Treatment of Generalized Anxiety Disorder

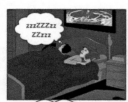

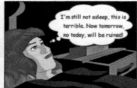

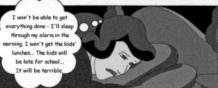

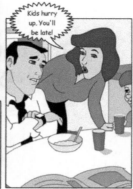

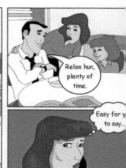

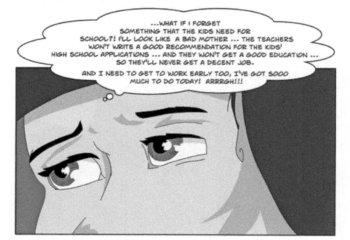

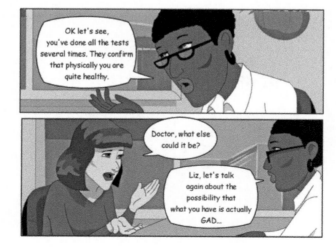

Treatment of Generalized Anxiety Disorder
Therapist Guides and Patient Manual

Gavin Andrews **MD**
Alison E. J. Mahoney **DPsych**
Megan J. Hobbs **PhD**
Margo R. Genderson **PhD**
Clinical Research Unit for Anxiety and Depression,
University of New South Wales at St Vincent's Hospital,
Sydney, Australia

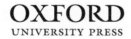

OXFORD
UNIVERSITY PRESS

OXFORD
UNIVERSITY PRESS

Great Clarendon Street, Oxford, OX2 6DP,
United Kingdom

Oxford University Press is a department of the University of Oxford.
It furthers the University's objective of excellence in research, scholarship,
and education by publishing worldwide. Oxford is a registered trade mark of
Oxford University Press in the UK and in certain other countries

© Oxford University Press 2016

The moral rights of the authors have been asserted

First Edition published in 2016

Impression: 1

Published in the United States of America by Oxford University Press
198 Madison Avenue, New York, NY 10016, United States of America

British Library Cataloguing in Publication Data

Data available

Library of Congress Control Number: 2015953851

ISBN 978-0-19-875884-6

Printed and bound by
CPI Group (UK) Ltd, Croydon, CR0 4YY

Oxford University Press makes no representation, express or implied, that the
drug dosages in this book are correct. Readers must therefore always check
the product information and clinical procedures with the most up-to-date
published product information and data sheets provided by the manufacturers
and the most recent codes of conduct and safety regulations. The authors and
the publishers do not accept responsibility or legal liability for any errors in the
text or for the misuse or misapplication of material in this work. Except where
otherwise stated, drug dosages and recommendations are for the non-pregnant
adult who is not breast-feeding

Links to third party websites are provided by Oxford in good faith and
for information only. Oxford disclaims any responsibility for the materials
contained in any third party website referenced in this work.

Preface

When scared, our hearts beat fast, we feel short of breath, we break out in a cold sweat, we tremble and shake, and less noticeably, our pupils dilate and attention focuses. These physical changes are adaptive and facilitate the fight or flight response. If the threat is imminent but not yet upon us, we feel aroused as we prepare to fight or flee, and the same body changes occur. In short, we are anxious and we have little capacity to attend to other matters.

If the threat is in the future, not imminent, we worry about it, thinking about ways to neutralize it. At best, this evokes images and thoughts of strategies whereby the problem can be solved, sometimes realistically and sometimes unrealistically. The focus of our worry is on appraisal of the threat and its solution, not on how the problem could escalate. Flight or fight arousal symptoms are present but the changes are commensurate with the degree of the immediate threat. We are worried, but we can put the worry aside to attend to everyday tasks.

Some people, in the absence of danger, see threats everywhere and worry day after day. As the reality of the threat is somewhat tenuous, the thought "what if I've forgotten something the kids need for school?" is justified by the worrying thought "I'll look like a bad mother" and so on, into the future, until the thought "and they'll never get a good job" seems unreasonable. In such people, the worrying thoughts are verbal, the excessive and uncontrollable escalation is future-oriented, physical arousal is chronic but constrained, and there is surprisingly little rehearsal of problem-solving strategies. Everyday tasks are interfered with. The behavior is not normal problem-oriented worrying.

People who are anxious and worry in a maladaptive way benefit from good, proactive treatment. That is the focus of this book. Across the board, the book will be valuable to all proponents of the scientist–practitioner model. We begin by tracing the history of generalized anxiety disorder (GAD). We then look at the effectiveness of pharmacological and psychological treatments, favoring the latter. In Chapter 4, we list contemporary models of GAD and explore new developments in cognitive behavior therapy. This chapter may be particularly applicable to the difficult-to-get-better patient. We then present a clinician's guide to treatment that covers assessment, formulation, and the beneficial and problematic steps in cognitive behavioral therapy. Finally, there is a patient treatment manual that can be used as a curriculum for individual or group therapy, or copied and provided to patients to work though on their own.

The first half of the book contains academic reviews that will be of most interest to researchers. The second half of the book contains practical advice that will be of most interest to clinicians and their patients. Now read on.

Disclaimer

GA and MH contributed to the DSM-5 proposals for the revision of the GAD classification. The views contained in this book are those of the authors and do not express the views or opinions of the American Psychiatric Association.

Contents

List of Figures

List of Tables and Forms

Tables

Forms

Chapter 1

DSM-5 generalized anxiety disorder: the product of an imperfect science

Introduction

Psychiatric classification is difficult. Nosologists need to strike a balance between utility and reliability, between tradition and validity, creating an evidence-based manual that withstands media sound bites. The generalized anxiety disorder (GAD) classification has proven more difficult than most. Introduced in the third edition of the *Diagnostic and Statistical Manual of Mental Disorders* (DSM-III) as a residual diagnosis, the GAD criteria had one of the lowest diagnostic reliabilities of the mood and anxiety disorders. The revised DSM-III breathed new life into the GAD criteria, identifying chronic apprehensive anxiety about multiple aspects of life as the defining feature of GAD. This innovation improved the reliability of GAD symptoms but concerns about reliability and validity of the diagnosis led some experts to suggest that GAD should be excluded from DSM-IV. This did not occur. After further revision in DSM-IV, the GAD criteria were established as an independent diagnosis. Some 30 years since the introduction of GAD in DSM-III, more recommendations were made to further improve the validity of the classification. Despite these recommendations and in the face of media skepticism about psychiatry as a science, none of these recommendations influenced the DSM-5 GAD classification. In this chapter, we trace the balancing act that has been the evolution of the GAD classification.

Creating a useful and reliable psychiatric classification

Clinicians need to use the DSM to distinguish between cases and non-cases of mental disorder and to distinguish between different types of mental disorder. Researchers need to use the classification for the same reason. Ideally, the way that the DSM defines these diagnostic boundaries is useful and reliable. Here, psychiatric classification becomes tricky. A useful classification is one that facilitates clinical and academic decision making and the communication of these decisions. Clinicians and academics should be able to read the DSM and understand the core clinical features of each disorder and recall these features when assessing cases. A reliable classification, however, is achieved by specifically defining the clinical features of the disorder by objective criteria. More often than not, the greater the specification, the greater the reliability of the diagnosis. Balancing utility with reliability is therefore a thin-edged sword. An unreliable psychiatric classification is useless. However, the more criteria that are used to define a disorder, the larger and more unwieldy the classification becomes. A psychiatric classification therefore needs to balance the need for useful diagnoses, which would include the minimum amount of detail needed to capture the core problem of each disorder, with reliable diagnoses, which use many criteria to specify disorders.

Generalized anxiety disorder (GAD) is an excellent example of how nosologists, who can improve diagnostic reliability, can also improve the utility of a diagnosis.

DSM-III

In DSM-III, GAD had no defining features. GAD had the lowest test–retest reliability estimate (other than simple phobia) with a kappa of 0.47 (Di Nardo et al., 1983). Inter-rater reliability estimates of the DSM-III GAD classification were only slightly higher, with fair agreement between experienced clinicians diagnosing a current episode of GAD (kappa = 0.57) (Barlow, 1985). Indeed, Barlow et al. (1986a) examined if GAD could be differentiated from depression and the other anxiety disorders based on the severity of patients' motor tension, autonomic hyperactivity, and vigilance scanning. No reliable distinctions were identified, and the authors concluded that there was little need to include GAD in the DSM as a residual diagnosis.

DSM-III-R

GAD was specified further in DSM-III-R. Repetitive thinking about the potential negative outcomes of future events concerning multiple aspects of life became the defining feature of the classification (Barlow et al., 1986b). Patients' anxiety and worry was identified as excessive, unrealistic, and difficult to control (Craske et al., 1989; Sanderson and Barlow, 1990). GAD was now classified as a chronic disorder (Barlow et al., 1986a). Eighteen associated symptoms were itemized.

Despite these changes to the classification, the reliability of DSM-III-R-defined GAD was still not ideal, yielding estimates comparable to DSM-III, and DSM-III-R GAD was associated with low test–retest lifetime estimates (kappa = 0.39) (Mannuzza et al., 1989). Inter-rater reliability was slightly better. There was an improved degree of inter-rater reliability for current cases of DSM-III-R-defined GAD (kappa of 0.56) (Williams et al., 1992) and for GAD as a principal diagnosis (kappa of 0.57) (Di Nardo et al., 1993). Although the diagnosis now had a unique and defining clinical feature, it was unclear why reliability estimates were not higher. Some experts hypothesized that it was difficult for clinicians to distinguish between the excessive worry of GAD and the obsessions of obsessive compulsive disorder (OCD). However, no inter-rater disagreements about whether patients' principal diagnosis was GAD or OCD could be identified (Brown et al., 1993).

Although the reasons for the relatively low reliability estimates remained elusive, the DSM-III-R GAD symptoms of worry could be assessed reliably. Sanderson and Barlow (1990) showed that individuals with GAD worried most about family, finances, work, and illness, and clinical assessments of the excessiveness and/or unrealistic nature of these worries had excellent reliability (kappa = 0.90) (Sanderson and Barlow, 1990). Craske and colleagues also found high agreement between raters about the types of things that individuals with GAD worry about (91.2%) (Craske et al., 1989). Nevertheless, DSM-III-R-defined GAD remained one of "the more conceptually challenging [diagnoses] in psychiatric nosology."

The DSM-III-R GAD diagnosis had fair reliability at best and, at worst, the classification was of little use, for clinicians or for academics. At least, this is what some clinicians and academics argued. The frequent co-occurrence of DSM-III-R-defined GAD with other mood and anxiety disorders further complicated the future of the GAD classification. Debate about merging GAD with another mood or anxiety disorder ensued (Brown, Barlow, and Liebowitz, 1994). Indeed, some DSM-IV Anxiety Disorders Work Group members suggested that the empirical basis of GAD was not sufficient to warrant the inclusion of GAD in DSM-IV. An alternative was floated. GAD could be removed from the main text of the DSM-IV and included in the Appendix.

DSM-IV

Despite this debate, GAD survived in DSM-IV. This decision was made because even though comorbidity with other anxiety and depressive disorders was common, there was a proportion of patients who met the diagnostic threshold for GAD but did not meet threshold criteria for an additional mood or anxiety disorder. In defense of the disorder, it was noted that disorders other than GAD also had high rates of comorbidity (Brawman-Mintzer et al., 1993; Brown and Barlow, 1992), and that GAD was associated with a different age of onset than other anxiety disorders (Brown, Barlow, and Liebowitz, 1994).

With the publication of DSM-IV, in which the long list of associated symptoms was reduced to a manageable number, the balance between reliability and utility came down on the side of utility. The reliability of the GAD classification may not have been excellent, but there appeared to be a group of patients whose core issue was excessive and generalized worry, and clinicians therefore saw a continued use for the classification.

The GAD classification may have avoided relegation to the Appendix of the DSM-IV but the classification did undergo a series of revisions before inclusion in DSM-IV. Excessive, difficult-to-control, and chronic generalized worry remained the defining feature of GAD. The classification however was shortened in other ways. The "unrealistic" criterion was omitted from the classification. The list of 18 associated symptoms was also cut and the six most frequently endorsed associated symptoms remained. There were, of course, people who endorsed the symptoms that were dropped. The job of a psychiatric classification is not to capture all variants of mental health problems. Instead, the classification needs to be pragmatic and to use the minimum number of symptoms to define each disorder, and to provide clinicians and researchers with sufficient detail to decide who meets the criteria for which disorder and who does not.

Reducing the number of symptoms in DSM-IV appears to have struck a good balance between detail and utility. The inter-rater reliability of the DSM-IV GAD classification trumped earlier classifications. There is good agreement about current (kappa = 0.65) and lifetime (kappa = 0.65) cases of DSM-IV GAD (Brown et al., 2001b; Lobbestael, Leurgans, and Arntz, 2011; Zanarini et al., 2000).

Balancing tradition and validity

Creating a useful and reliable classification may be difficult, but creating a reliable classification that is valid continues to challenge nosologists. The frequent co-occurrence of GAD with other mood and anxiety disorders, and what this co-occurrence means for the validity of the diagnosis, was a ubiquitous theme in the early GAD literature. It is more common in clinical practice to see people who experience GAD with other disorders than as a sole diagnosis (Brown and Barlow, 1992; Brown et al., 2001a). GAD also co-occurs with mood and other anxiety disorders in the community, albeit to a lesser degree than in clinical samples. Two thirds of current cases of GAD will experience at least one additional diagnosis (Hunt, Issakidis, and Andrews, 2002). Comorbidity is not reserved to GAD. All mood and anxiety disorders co-occur more often than not (Hettema, Prescott, and Kendler, 2003; Moffitt et al., 2007; Pine et al., 1998). More than half of the general population who experience a common mental disorder in their lives will experience more than one mental disorder (Kessler et al., 2005a; Slade et al., 2009).

To put fears about comorbidity and GAD to rest, the questions were not: does GAD co-occur with other disorders and is GAD secondary to them? Instead, the real questions to be answered were: are there people who meet criteria for GAD and regard it as more distressing and disabling than the other disorders, and are there people who meet criteria for GAD that have no other mental disorder and have significant distress and impairment as a result? There is, and they do (Kessler et al., 2002; Wittchen et al., 2000). So perhaps co-occurrence of GAD with other disorders should not have been a problem for the GAD classification. Hindsight is always 20/20.

Psychiatric classification may be difficult but Barlow, Brown, and their DSM-IV Work Group contemporaries crafted increasingly useful and reliable criteria for GAD. Specifically, the evolving classification has progressively facilitated clinical distinctions to be made between GAD and adaptive worry, and between GAD and other mood and anxiety disorders. Academics have also been able to grow the empirical basis about the prevalence of GAD and about the risk factors and clinical correlates of the disorder.

DSM-IV-defined GAD is common. One in twenty adults experience GAD in their lives (4.1% to 6.0%) (Grant et al., 2005; Kessler et al., 2005b; Kessler and Wittchen, 2002; McEvoy, Grove, and Slade, 2011) and half of these adults report that they have experienced GAD in the past year (1.5% to 3.6%) (Carter et al., 2001; Hunt, Issakidis, and Andrews, 2002; Kessler, 2005a). Less data are available with respect to the population prevalence of GAD in childhood and adolescence. Estimates range between 0.8% and 2.2% for lifetime estimates and between 0.5% and 1.1% for past-year estimates (Kessler et al., 2012a, b; Wittchen, Nelson, and Lachner, 1998). The prevalence varies by gender and age. Females are twice as likely to experience GAD as males (Carter et al., 2001; Grant et al., 2005; Maier et al., 2000). GAD peaks in prevalence in middle age and declines in prevalence in the later years of life (Carter et al., 2001; Grant et al., 2005; Hunt, Issakidis, and Andrews, 2002; Kessler et al., 2005b).

GAD may be common but, as with most psychiatric disorders, the necessary and sufficient causes of GAD are not known. What is known is that one third of the liability to develop GAD is under genetic control (Hettema, Prescott, and Kendler, 2004; Kendler et al., 1994, 2003) and that the within-familial environment does not contribute substantially to developing GAD (0–4% of the liability) (Hettema et al., 2006; Kendler et al., 1992). This means that individual non-family environmental factors are the greatest predictor of GAD, and these are only modestly related to those factors associated with experiencing major depressive disorder (MDD) (Hettema et al., 2006; Hettema, Prescott, and Kendler, 2004; Kendler et al., 1995, 2003, 2007). The special environmental triggers for GAD, however, are unclear. Childhood adversities are known to increase the likelihood of the development and persistence of all of the common mental disorders (Green et al., 2010; McLaughlin et al., 2010) but are neither necessary nor sufficient for, or specific to, GAD.

Some dose relationship between environmental factors and GAD may explain the relatively late age of first onset of GAD, which is in the early 30s (Grant et al., 2005; Kessler et al., 2005b). GAD may begin early in life but manifest as an anxious or neurotic temperament which, when paired with environmental triggers, results in acute episodes of anxiety (Akiskal, 1998; Kagan and Snidman, 1999). These acute periods of anxiety may increase in duration across the lifespan and, therefore, people who do not meet the criteria for their first episode of DSM-IV-defined GAD until their 30s may have experienced increasing periods of anxiety and worry prior to this (Kessler and Wittchen, 2002; Starvcevic and Bogojevic, 1999). This hypothesis is consistent with the slow waxing and waning course of GAD (Angst et al., 2009; Ballenger et al., 2001). GAD is characterized by periods of worrying that tend to last for months or years rather than days or hours (Grant et al., 2005; Yonkers et al., 2003).

Despite the chronic course of GAD, less than half of people who experience GAD seek treatment. Those who seek treatment wait more than ten years after the onset (Wang et al., 2005). Even then, treatment tends to be sought for comorbid somatic panic and depressive symptoms rather than anxiety (Judd et al., 1998; Kessler and Wittchen, 2002). A low number of people with GAD seek treatment from specialized mental health services, preferring to consult primary care physicians rather than psychologists or psychiatrists, and GAD is the most common anxiety disorder in primary care (Maier et al., 2000; Üstun and Sartorius, 1995; Wittchen, 2002).

The balance that nosologists have iteratively struck between the reliability, utility, and validity of the classification has delineated the prevalence and some of the risk factors and clinical correlates of GAD. These data show that GAD can be differentiated from other disorders. We said that, at one level, these data support the validity of the

GAD diagnosis. However, at another level, the traditional approach to classifying GAD as a categorical disorder may be limited. There are increasing structural data that show that many different disorders are experienced to different degrees. The diagnostic boundaries between adaptive cognitions and behaviors and mental disorders are porous. Most mental disorders exist as continuous phenotypes; most mental disorders are dimensional. For instance, people can be sad, but fleetingly so. People can endorse only a few of the symptoms of MDD and be below threshold, and those above threshold can have mild, moderate, or severe MDD. Exactly the same dimension occurs in GAD, from short periods of excessive worry to chronic and excessive worry that produces significant distress and impairment. The use of diagnostic symptoms and thresholds to define disorders do not, therefore, identify discrete diseases that are independent of healthy and adaptive cognitions and behaviors (Kendell and Jablensky, 2003). Instead, DSM symptoms index varying degrees of diagnostic severity; the diagnostic criteria define the point at which the disorder is identified as likely to require treatment.

No structural data have examined the relative validity of treating GAD as a categorical or dimensional phenotype. However, people worry to varying degrees (Ruscio, Borkovec, and Ruscio, 2001) and, as a core feature of GAD, this suggests GAD may also be dimensional. Epidemiological data about GAD suggest as much. If subthreshold and threshold cases of GAD were discrete, then it would be expected that these groups of individuals would be qualitatively distinct with respect to their risk factors, clinical correlates, and/or associated disability. However, epidemiological studies that have examined the risk factors and correlates of subthreshold and threshold cases of GAD show that these groups of individuals are not qualitatively distinct. Instead, individuals who endorse all the diagnostic criteria for GAD except, for example, that their anxiety was not excessive or that their symptoms lasted for less than six months, are similar with respect to risk and clinical correlates to individuals who endorsed all the criteria for GAD (Angst et al., 2009; Bienvenu, Nestadt, and Eaton, 1998; Lee et al., 2009; Maier et al., 2000; Ruscio et al., 2005; Slade and Andrews, 2001). These data suggest that there is a degree of continuity between subthreshold and threshold cases of GAD. The balance that the DSM strikes between its categorical heritage and what the data say is convenient but may be misleading.

The traditional categorical approach in psychiatric classification of identifying distinct types of disorder is also problematic. Contrary to the traditional notions of psychiatric validity (Robins and Guze, 1970), the data have simply not proven that mental disorders are independent from each other. Instead, the comorbidity problem keeps rearing its head. There are consistent patterns that characterize the co-occurrence of the common mental disorders. For example, individuals who experience a unipolar mood or anxiety disorder are more likely to experience other anxiety disorders and mood disorders than substance use disorders, and people who experience substance use disorders are more likely to experience multiple substance use or conduct disorders than mood and anxiety disorders (Kessler et al., 2012b; Teesson, Slade, and Mills, 2009).

Numerous hypotheses about the reasons for diagnostic comorbidity exist. For example:

1. Comorbidity could result by chance.
2. The occurrence of one diagnosis could increase the risk of developing additional diagnoses.
3. Comorbidity could indicate that the respective disorders share a common diathesis.
4. Comorbidity could be a result of incorrectly lumping and splitting symptoms that index a shared pathology (Andrews, 1996; Hyman, 2007; Maser and Patterson, 2002).

Given that diagnoses co-occur at rates far exceeding chance levels, the first explanation is unlikely. There are, however, robust data that show that two latent factors explain the co-occurrence of the common mental disorders: the *internalizing* and the *externalizing* factors (Cox, Clara, and Enns, 2002; Krueger, 1999b; Krueger et al., 1998, 2003; Krueger and Markon, 2006; Lahey et al., 2008; Markon, 2010; Slade and Watson, 2006; Vollebergh et al., 2001). The internalizing factor explains the co-occurrence of the unipolar mood and the anxiety disorders. The externalizing factor explains the co-occurrence of the substance use and antisocial disorders.

Some studies have also found support for a division within the internalizing disorders, with the co-occurrence of GAD, MDD, dysthymia, and post-traumatic stress disorder (PTSD) explained by an *anxious/misery* subfacet of the internalizing factor, whereas the co-occurrence of panic and some of the phobic disorders is explained by reference to a *fear* subfacet of the internalizing factor (Krueger, 1999b; Slade and Watson, 2006). There is robust support for this internalizing–externalizing factor structure of the common mental disorders across age groups (Eaton, Krueger, and Oltmanns, 2011; Krueger et al., 1998; Lahey et al., 2008), ethnicities (Eaton et al., 2012), and countries (Fergusson, Horwood, and Boden, 2006; Kessler et al., 2005a; Krueger et al., 2003; Slade and Watson, 2006; Vollebergh et al., 2001). The internalizing–externalizing model of the occurrence of the common mental disorders has also been extended to explain the occurrence of psychotic-like experiences (Laurens et al., 2012; Wright et al., 2013). As well as explaining the phenotypic covariance of the unipolar mood and anxiety disorders, the internalizing factor explains the genotypic covariation and the shared environmental risk factors of these disorders (Hettema, Neale, and Kendler, 2001; Kendler et al., 2011; Kendler, Davis, and Kessler, 1997; Kendler et al., 2003). This common genetic covariation also overlaps with the genetic risk of being neurotic (Hettema et al., 2006). These patterns of comorbidity, risk factors, and clinical correlates challenge the validity of the notion that the DSM is "carving nature at its joints" and identifying discrete diseases by applying the categorical approach to classification (Kendell and Jablensky, 2003).

In an attempt to bring tradition into accordance with reality, proposals were made to reconfigure the DSM-5 chapters. Based on the risk factor similarities between many disorders, five disorder chapters were proposed for DSM-5: the neurodevelopmental, neurocognitive, internalizing, externalizing, and psychotic-like disorders (Andrews et al., 2009a, b; Carpenter et al., 2009; Goldberg et al., 2009; Krueger and South, 2009; Sachdev et al., 2009). To some extent, the organization of DSM-5 follows this arrangement (American Psychiatric Association, 2013). The important relationships within the internalizing disorders and within the externalizing disorders, and between both clusters of disorders, are explicitly described in the manual (Regier, Kuhl, and Kupfer, 2013). Balancing validity with tradition is a slow incremental progression that requires caution and ongoing efforts.

Designing a classification that is valid but withstands media sound bites

DSM-5's recognition of the internalizing disorders shows that, in some instances, data prevail. At other times, the data do not. The DSM-5 Anxiety, Obsessive-Compulsive Spectrum, Post-traumatic, and Dissociative Disorders Work Group (the "Work Group") was charged with the responsibility of reclassifying GAD. Recommendations were made on the basis of reviewing the data pertaining to the reliability and validity of the DSM-IV GAD classification as well as the effect on DSM-IV cases if specific diagnostic criteria were omitted or introduced to the GAD classification in DSM-5 (Andrews et al., 2010a).

The Work Group found that omitting the excessiveness criterion could improve the reliability of the diagnosis (Wittchen et al., 1998) and such a classification would identify the same type of patients as the DSM-IV classification with respect to their socio-demographics, treatment-seeking behaviors, and familiality of anxiety disorders (Beesdo-Baum et al., 2011; Ruscio et al., 2005). However, the Group proposed that the excessive criterion should continue to be a defining feature of GAD in DSM-5 because there was a lack of evidence that supported the inclusion of a different defining feature and the traditional connection of excessive worry with the GAD classification.

Andrews et al. (2010a) also recommended that the "multiple circumstances" criterion should be retained. This was because no data have emerged since the inclusion of this feature in DSM-III-R to dispute the use of generalized anxious apprehension as the defining feature of GAD. Instead, there has been robust support for Barlow et al.'s (1986b) and Craske et al.'s (1989) findings that GAD patients worry about many aspects of their life. For instance, Roemer and colleagues examined whether individuals who met threshold criteria for GAD worry more and worry about different things than individuals who do not meet threshold criteria for GAD (Roemer, Molina, and Borkovec,

1997). Individuals with GAD were found to experience more generalized worry and worry more about family/interpersonal and miscellaneous topics such as minor matters and routine daily activities than individuals without GAD (Roemer, Molina, and Borkovec, 1997). GAD patients also worry about more topics, particularly interpersonal relationships, finances, religion/ politics/ environment, and 'daily hassles' than patients with social phobia (Hoyer et al., 2001).

The Work Group also examined the duration of the GAD classification. Here, the data in favor of revision were strong. The six-month criterion was introduced in DSM-III-R to reflect the chronicity of GAD, and research suggested that it did not set the threshold for the disorder too high. While there is a group of worriers who experience their generalized anxious expectation for more than six months (Barlow et al., 1986a), a longer duration criterion has been shown to reduce the reliability of the diagnosis (from a kappa of 0.70 with a one-month duration to a kappa of 0.45 with a six-month duration (Wittchen et al., 1998). Numerous studies have also shown that a classification with a lower duration threshold (e.g., one month or three months) would identify respondents with similar symptom severity and clinical impairment to the current six-month threshold (Angst et al., 2006; Kessler et al., 2005c; Maier et al., 2000). A lower duration threshold would also identify individuals with similar socio-demographics (Angst et al., 2006; Bienvenu, Nestadt, and Eaton, 1998; Kessler et al., 2005c), mean age of onset (Lee et al., 2009), familial risk of GAD (Beesdo-Baum et al., 2011; Kendler et al., 1994), and comorbidity profiles (Beesdo-Baum et al., 2011; Kessler et al., 2005c; Lee et al., 2009) to the current six-month threshold. Based on these data, Andrews et al. (2010a) recommended that the six-month duration criterion be reduced to three months.

In contrast to the substantive literature that has developed around the "excessive," "multiple life events," and duration criteria of the GAD classification, few data were available to the DSM-5 GAD reviewers about the "difficulty to control" criterion. The combined clinical expertise of the Work Group converged on the conclusion that there is a substantial overlap between the "excessive" and "difficult to control" constructs. This observation, paired with the finding from the Early Developmental

Stages of Psychopathology Study that only 4% of children with GAD who endorsed all of the other DSM-IV criteria for GAD reported that their worry was excessive but was still controllable (Beesdo-Baum et al., 2011), supported the omission of the "difficulty to control" criterion in DSM-5. If "excessive" and "difficult to control" are overlapping concepts, and the former is difficult to judge reliably, then perhaps the latter could be the best defining criteria.

In DSM-IV, the 18 associated symptoms used to define DSM-III-R GAD were reduced to six symptoms. This revision was based on data that showed that the six associated symptoms retained in DSM-IV were the most frequently endorsed by patients with GAD. With the object of improving the discriminant validity of the GAD classification, Andrews et al. (2010a) proposed that of the six DSM-IV-associated symptoms, only two, muscle tension and restlessness, should be included in DSM-5, and that the other four DSM-IV-associated symptoms should be omitted from the classification. The DSM-IV-associated symptoms "restless or feeling keyed up or on edge" and "muscle tension" are specific to GAD. The other four are not, and three are restatements of symptoms found in major depression. This proposal is supported by data that show that reducing the number of associated symptoms in the GAD diagnosis has little effect on the prevalence of the disorder. For instance, secondary analyses of the first Australian National Survey of Mental Health were conducted to assess the effect of deleting the associated symptom criterion (e.g., criterion C) on the prevalence of the disorder. It was found that without any associated symptoms, the prevalence of 12-month GAD increased by only 4.2%. The symptoms that were endorsed by most individuals with GAD were restless (88%), keyed up or on edge (89%), fatigue (79%), difficulty concentrating (82%), irritable (82%), and muscle tension (59%). If, however, deleting all of the associated symptoms has little effect on the prevalence of the disorder and would increase the specificity of the disorder, there seems little point in retaining the non-specific associated symptom criteria (i.e., fatigue, difficulty concentrating, sleep disturbance, and irritability).

The DSM-5 Work Group also proposed the introduction of behavioral avoidance criteria, which would be consistent with the use of this type of criteria to define the other anxiety disorders. Moreover, avoidance behaviors are directly observable and reflect the leading cognitive behavioral models of GAD that:

(i)   patients with GAD avoid events that could have negative consequences for themselves and/or their loved ones

(ii) patients spend a marked amount of time preparing for future events, the outcomes of which they worry about

(iii) patients procrastinate in order to avoid the potential negative outcomes of future events

(iv) patients with GAD seek reassurance excessively to reduce their immediate anxiety (Andrews et al., 2010a).

Following the submission of the Work Group's proposals to the DSM-5 Scientific Committee, the DSM-5 Field Trials were conducted. The purpose of the Field Trials was to examine the test–retest reliability and convergent validity of the Work Group proposals using a multi-site stratified sampling design (Clarke et al., 2013; Regier et al., 2013). The DSM-5 GAD proposals were tested at one site using 44 psychiatric outpatients who completed both assessments and were associated with an intra-class kappa of 0.20 (Clarke et al., 2013; Regier, 2013). No symptom-level reliability data have been published. This level of test–retest reliability is not acceptable. Like any other research, the Field Trials have their methodological limits. The DSM-5 Field Trials did not assess the influence of the proposals on prevalence or validity (Dayle Jones, 2012). This is unfortunate given that the proposals were aimed at improving the validity of GAD. Additional evaluations of the effect of the proposals on the prevalence of diagnoses and the validity of the proposals are therefore essential to maintaining and potentially improving the validity of GAD.

Two additional studies have been conducted that have assessed the impact of the DSM-5 GAD proposals. Andrews et al. (2010a) examined the effect of omitting the criteria outlined in the DSM-5 proposals in a nationally representative epidemiologic survey of community dwelling adults, and also investigated the combined effect of all of the proposed revisions on cases in a clinical sample. Reducing the duration criterion increased the prevalence of GAD, whereas revising the associated symptoms and adding behavioral symptoms reduced the prevalence of the diagnosis. With all the new options implemented, the prevalence of the diagnosis rose by 9%, which means that the prevalence of 3% would rise to 3.27% and would be associated with similar levels of distress and impairment as DSM-IV cases.

In another study conducted by Comer, Pincus, and Hofmann (2012), the effect of omitting the non-specific-associated symptoms from the GAD classification in a treatment-seeking sample of anxious youths was examined. Reducing the associated symptom list to include only restlessness and muscle tension meant that 10.9% of youths who met the threshold criteria for DSM-IV GAD would not meet the proposed DSM-5 criteria for a diagnosis, even though they had similar clinical severity, symptoms, and functioning to those who continued to meet the criteria for GAD. Comer and colleagues concluded that "losing" 10% of cases would not be a satisfactory outcome. However, a 90% rate of agreement is an excellent rate of concordance between the two criteria sets. In light of the limitations of the DSM-5 Field Trials and the burden attributable to the GAD classification, further empirical research into the combined effect of the DSM-5 proposals is essential.

Throughout this chapter, we have discussed the balancing acts that nosologists face. Nosologists responsible for GAD in DSM-5 made recommendations based on available evidence. None of these proposals influenced the DSM-5 GAD criteria. There are two explanations for this. The American Psychiatric Association, in its balancing act of utility and reliability, and tradition and validity, favored reliability and tradition. There was considerable political and media pressure to keep the status quo. Plans for the DSM-5 were always ambitious, and ambitious empirical exercises that move away from tradition are never easy and often face opposition. In academia, we engage in discourse in peer-reviewed journals. This has been the case since the start of psychiatry as a science. Nosologists have, therefore, traditionally faced opposition by other academics and clinicians in scientific journals.

DSM-5 is a product, however, of a different time, compared to DSM-III. We now live in a digital age. Everyone has an opinion. People share these opinions on social media sites, such as Twitter and blogs. The 24-hour media cycle operates in sound bites. Somehow, through this digital discourse, opinions that are scientific and non-scientific, or data-driven and opinion-based, have become increasingly equal. The American Psychiatric Association appointed experts who had an extensive track record in the identification, epidemiology, and treatment of anxiety disorders to make proposals for the reclassification of GAD. This combined expertise guided their review. Media outlets and DSM dissidents argued that the DSM-5 process, in general, was pathologizing normality. GAD was an easy target. Everybody worries. Not everyone understands how GAD is different from worry. Ignorance breeds hostility and can be easily manipulated into sound bites. The media may not be perfect but neither is expert consensus. Nothing about psychiatry is perfect but it is a profession. It is a science, and the rules of this science are not easily expressed in sound bites. The outputs of an imperfect science should by no means be trusted without scrutiny. However, science should be scrutinized by the informed and in the correct forums. The proposals for all of the DSM-5 disorders were scrutinized. They were scrutinized by the American Psychiatric Association, the external academics who reviewed the proposals before they were published in scientific journals, and by the media—and the result was a continuation of DSM-IV criteria for GAD in DSM-5.

Conclusions

DSM-5 is still new, but much of the controversy that preceded publication has died away. Nonetheless, as we progress to DSM-6, we know that nosolgists will continue to try to strike a balance between utility, reliability, validity, and the political process. This balance may be difficult to achieve and require patience, but a good balance can only benefit the health of patients who experience GAD.

Questions for future research

Is the title the problem?

People who meet the criteria for GAD are not "generalizedly" anxious, and do not display the physical symptoms of anxiety all the time.

Instead, they worry and anticipate difficulties, but the physical manifestations are limited. If the disorder was called "major worry disorder" would recognition and treatment be more reliable and valid?

Is GAD dimensional in nature?

GAD has traditionally been conceptualized and classified as a categorical disorder. This approach to classification assumes that GAD is qualitatively distinct from adaptive apprehensive expectation and other disorders. The data suggest that this approach is not valid. Structural examinations that test the relative fit of continuous and categorical models of GAD are needed to make firm conclusions in this area of research. No such data exist for GAD.

Why are some people more likely than others to experience GAD?

Females are more likely than males, and the middle aged are more likely than the young and the elderly to experience GAD. Caucasians are more likely than non-Caucasians to experience GAD. Why do these prevalence differences occur? Is the DSM biased towards specific groups? For instance, do females experience GAD in a different way to males, and does the increased prevalence of GAD in females occur because the DSM is more closely aligned with the female experience? Do psychosocial or biological factors that differ between groups explain these prevalence differences? Little work has been conducted around these important questions.

What is the relationship between "excessive" and "difficult to control" apprehensive expectation?

There were scant data to guide the DSM-5 Work Group in their revision of the difficult to control criterion. Clinical consensus suggested that there was a large overlap between the excessive and difficult to control criteria. Do data support this conclusion? Moreover, how should these two criteria be operationalized in practice? For instance, is it the clinician or the patient who should determine whether the patient's anxiety is excessive? Is it the amount of time spent worrying that is important to diagnostic assessment? Different ways of operationalizing these criteria have been conducted in the past but what is needed is data around the relative reliability, utility, and validity of these different approaches for predicting clinical change.

What areas of behavioral avoidance are most relevant to GAD?

Various forms of avoidance are reported in all anxiety disorders. Currently, there is a lack of standardized measures to assess avoidance in GAD. Such measures are needed to explore which avoidance behaviors (if any) are most pertinent to GAD and which are transdiagnostic. Identifying core forms of avoidance may help to enhance current treatments, as well as have implications for the conceptualization and diagnosis of GAD.

Chapter 2

Generalized anxiety disorder assessment measures

Introduction

The DSM-5 is 947 pages long. Since 2013, we have been able to diagnose more than 200 disorders. Each disorder is defined using lists of symptoms. The specific symptoms that are used to define each disorder and the number and/or combination of symptoms that are used to distinguish cases from non-cases are identified by consensus expert judgment based on a review of the empirical data (Regier et al., 2009). Most disorders include three or more criteria, with each criterion including several pieces of information. Therefore, a conservative estimate of the number of different pieces of information that the DSM includes is 1200. Indeed, the DSM includes many more pieces of information than this. For instance, post-traumatic stress disorder spans four pages of the new text. No clinician or researcher can retain this level of detail. Even if we were to silo the DSM disorders into large groups based on their risk factors, clinical correlates, and who treated these disorders—aged care services treat neurocognitive disorders, disability services treat neurodevelopmental disorders, psychiatrists focus on schizophrenia and bipolar disorders, psychologists and primary physicians treat mood and anxiety disorders, and drug and alcohol services treat substance use disorders—it is still unrealistic to believe that most clinicians and researchers can cite, verbatim, all of the inclusion and exclusion criteria for the disorders for which they have responsibility.

Structured diagnostic interviews

What are we then to do for clinicians and researchers who need to identify cases of GAD? The job of diagnosing using the explicit DSM criteria is easier for academics than for non-academic clinicians and physicians. Researchers, more often than not, have diagnostic instruments of known psychometric properties at their disposal. Most studies focus on one or a limited number of disorders. These diagnostic measures map neatly onto the diagnostic classifications and provide the user with a diagnosis.

Composite International Diagnostic Interview

The gold standard for epidemiological research is the World Mental Health Composite International Diagnostic Interview (CIDI 3.0) (Kessler and Üstun, 2004). The CIDI has been used as the base diagnostic instrument in the US National Comorbidity Survey Replication (Kessler and Merikangas, 2004) and its adolescent supplement (Kessler et al., 2009), National Latino and Asian American Study (NLAAS) (Alegria et al., 2004), National Survey of American Life (Jackson et al., 2004), the World Mental Health Surveys of 28 countries (Kessler et al., 2006), and the 2007 Australian National Survey of Mental Health and Well Being (Slade et al., 2009). The CIDI 3.0 is fully structured, is organized into modules, and uses a stem-probe interview format. Clinical reappraisal studies generally provide good concordance of CIDI diagnoses with blinded clinical diagnoses (Kessler et al., 1998; Wittchen, Zhao, and Kessler, 1994).

Anxiety Disorders Interview Schedule

What the CIDI is to epidemiologists, the Anxiety Disorders Interview Schedule for DSM-IV (ADIS-IV) (Brown, Di Nardo, and Barlow, 1994; Di Nardo, Brown, and Barlow, 1994) is to clinicians. Slightly less structured than the CIDI, clinicians use the ADIS to rate the frequency/intensity of patients' GAD symptoms on a nine-point scale, where higher scores indicate more intense anxiety and associated symptoms. The ADIS-IV has shown good agreement between independent raters for a principal diagnosis of current GAD (kappa = 0.67) and for a lifetime

GAD diagnosis (kappa = 0.65) (Brown et al., 2001b). Evidence of construct validity, including discriminant and convergent validity, has also been demonstrated (Brown, Chorpita, and Barlow, 1998).

Structured Clinical Interview for Axis I DSM-IV Disorders

Similarly, clinicians use the Structured Clinical Interview for Axis I DSM-IV Disorders (SCID) (First et al., 1997), which is less structured than the ADIS. GAD symptoms are scored on a four-point scale (inadequate information, absent, subthreshold, and threshold). Two studies have assessed the reliability of the DSM-IV SCID-I GAD module. Zanarini et al. (2000) examined the concordance of the SCID-I with the Diagnostic Interview for DSM-IV Personality Disorders and found good inter-rater agreement, with a kappa of 0.63, although the SCID-I had only fair test–retest reliability, with an estimated kappa of 0.44 (Zanarini et al., 2000). Lobbestael, Leurgans, and Arntz (2011) found higher test–retest reliability of the SCID-I than Zanarini and colleagues, following interviews with 151 patients. Fair agreement was found between the two raters regarding GAD (kappa = 0.75) (Lobbestael, Leurgans, and Arntz 2011).

Symptom measures

Rarely do non-academic clinicians or physicians use or have the time to administer a slew of diagnostic instruments. In the time constraints of typical clinical practice, they must then look for patients' core diagnostic issues. Two good self-report questionnaires are the Penn State Worry Questionnaire (PSWQ) (Molina and Borkovec, 1994) and the Generalized Anxiety Disorder-7 (GAD-7) (Spitzer et al., 2006).

Penn State Worry Questionnaire

The PSWQ is a self-report measure of 16 items which are rated on a five-point likert scale (e.g., "not at all typical of me" to "very typical of me") with five items reverse scored. A total score of the excessive, uncontrollability, and pervasive nature of the respondents' worry is calculated by summing the 16 items. The PSWQ has excellent internal consistency (α = 0.85–0.93) (Meyer et al., 1990; Molina and Borkovec, 1994) and can be used to discriminate between GAD and other anxiety disorders and individuals without disorders (Brown, Antony, and Barlow, 1992). The PSWQ has good test–retest reliability in undergraduate students across a two- to ten-week period (Meyer et al., 1990; Molina and Borkovec, 1994; Stöber, 1998) and is sensitive to change across six- and 12-week interventions (Borkovec and Costello, 1993).

Generalized Anxiety Disorder-7

The GAD-7 is a brief self-report screener for GAD that measures symptoms over the past two weeks. It can be downloaded from the internet, at no cost. The respondent is asked "over the last two weeks, how often have you been bothered by the following problems?" and each symptom is measured on a four-point likert scale (0 = not at all; 1 = several days; 2 = more than half the days; 3 = nearly every day). A total score is derived by summing the responses to the seven items. For patients in primary care, a score of ten is suggestive of a diagnosis of GAD (Spitzer et al., 2006). The internal consistency of the seven items is excellent (α = 0.92) as is the test–retest reliability of the instrument (intra-class correlation = 0.83). There is also excellent agreement between GAD-7 total scores and a GAD diagnosis from an interview with a mental health professional (clinical psychologist or senior psychiatric social worker) (intra-class correlation coefficient [ICC] = 0.83). Increasing GAD-7 total scores predicted increasing subscale scores on the 20-item Short Form Health Survey (SF-20), but were more related to mental health (α = 0.75) than the other subscales (e.g., social functioning, general health perceptions, bodily pain, role functioning, and physical functioning) (Spitzer et al., 2006).

In short, even time-restricted clinicians and physicians can diagnose likely cases of GAD in an empirically validated way.

Chapter 3

Treatment effectiveness

Pharmacological treatments

For 20 years, benzodiazepines—valium through to alprazolam—seemed the treatment for people who were identified as having generalized anxiety disorder (GAD), that is, people who were far too anxious and troubled by the somatic symptoms of their anxiety. Benzodiazepines were classified as anxiolytic medications, and they did have a short-term effect on anxiety, whatever its cause. This approach seemed logical. Prescribing benzodiazepines is, however, no longer the logical choice, and these drugs are no more a recommended treatment for GAD which, after all, is not characterized by being too anxious but, instead, by continuing worry. Due mainly to the adverse effects generated by these compounds, such as tolerance and dependency, and cognitive and motor disorders manifested in poor work or by traffic accidents, opinion has shifted towards the use of safer and more effective medications and to the use of psychological treatments (Martin et al., 2007).

A review completed for a NICE (National Institute of Clinical Excellence–UK) guideline on the management of GAD in adults concluded that because of dependence, benzodiazepines "did not appear to be an appropriate medication for use with people with GAD who often require long term treatment". However, escitalopram, paroxetine, and sertraline (SSRIs: selective serotonin reuptake inhibitors); duloxetine and venlafaxine (SNRIs: serotonin and norepinephrine reuptake inhibitors); and pregabalin (an anticonvulsant) were considered to have "sufficient clinical effectiveness data and acceptable harm-to-benefit ratios" to be considered as first-line pharmacological treatments for GAD (NICE, 2011). Sertraline was judged to have the highest probability of overall response and the best cost-effectiveness profile, dominating all other treatment options. The guideline concluded that "pharmacological interventions should only be routinely offered to people who have not benefitted from psychological interventions."

In the last ten years, there have been a number of meta-analytic reviews of the efficacy of medications in GAD. Mitte et al. (2005) reviewed 48 studies. Two thirds of the replicated studies were of benzodiazepines, one quarter of azapirones, and an eighth of SSRI/SNRIs. The mean effect size (ES) superiority over pill placebo control in the reduction of anxiety was 0.33, and no differences in efficacy between classes of medication were reported. Mitte (2005) then added 19 studies of psychological treatments, mainly cognitive behavior therapy (CBT) or behavior therapy (BT) versus wait-list controls, and compared the results with the use of medication versus pill placebo from the previous paper. Conclusions were hampered because, while both control groups accommodated natural history, the pill placebo added the moralizing effect of being in treatment, hence the pre–post change in the pill placebo group used in the medication studies was larger than the change in the wait-list control groups used in the CBT studies. Gould et al. (1997) were the first to highlight this problem, but Mitte was able to use a complex method to adjust the data and concluded that, while the improvement with pharmacotherapy was probably larger than that with CBT, CBT was likely to be preferred to medication because of better adherence. More recently, Goncalves and Byrne (2012) reviewed the treatment of GAD in older adults. Treatment effect sizes for pharmacological (0.32) and psychological (0.33) therapy were identical, exactly matching Mitte's original finding.

Hidalgo, Tupler, and Davidson (2007) reviewed 21 placebo-controlled trials of medications for GAD using the Hamilton Anxiety Rating Scale (HAM-A) change from baseline to endpoint after a mean of eight weeks. HAM-A change scores in people allocated to placebo were considerable, and the mean ES superiority of medication over placebo was 0.39. The authors found differences between the classes of medication (pregabalin ES = 0.50, antihistamine 0.45, SNRIs 0.42, benzodiazepine 0.38, SSRIs 0.36, azapirones 0.17), with no differences in effect size between the azapirones and placebo. Effect sizes were stronger in children than adults. Baldwin, Waldman, and Allgulander (2011) provide a review of RCTs (randomized controlled trials) and Baldwin et al. (2011) included 27 trials in a probabilistic meta-analysis of drug treatments for GAD. Confining attention to drugs that were the subject of three or more studies, duloxetine, followed by sertraline, produced the greatest response; escitalopram, followed by venlafaxine, the greatest remission; and sertraline, followed by pregabalin, the greatest tolerability.

In a Cochrane review of azapirones (Chessick et al., 2006), 36 placebo-controlled trials were studied on the basis of changes in the Clinical Global Impressions Scale. Azapirones were superior to placebo but less effective than benzodiazepines, consistent with the Hidalgo, Tupler, and Davidson review (2007). Studying the benefit of second-generation antipsychotics, LaLonde and Van Lieshout (2011) concluded that the addition of these drugs in treatment-refractory GAD did not produce any benefit. The second-generation antipsychotic quetiapine, however, when used as a primary treatment, was more efficacious than placebo, but is probably not indicated because tolerability was low. Finally, Boschen (2011) examined seven trials of pregabalin compared to placebo, measured with the HAM-A. The mean ES superiority over placebo was 0.35 and the degree of response was strongly correlated (0.95) with the degree of placebo response in the same study, a finding that casts doubt on the specificity of the response to pregabalin.

In summary, medication is not a strong treatment for GAD (see Box 3.1). An ES superiority over control group of 0.35, the average of studies reviewed here, is consistent with the number needed to treat for one to recover being five (NNT = 5). NICE considered that medications should only be used when psychological treatments have failed. SSRI/SNRIs, the most commonly prescribed medications, have been associated with serious side-effects (e.g., sexual difficulties, dependence) in as many as half, and with a risk of agitation (as does pregabalin), on occasions leading to suicide in the young, and in falls leading to death in the old, so that the number needed to treat to produce harm is of the order of two (NNH = 2) (Gotzsche, 2014).

> Box 3.1 **Summary: medication for GAD (NNT = 5; NNH = 2)**
>
> ◆ Benzodiazepines should not be prescribed for the treatment of GAD due to adverse side-effects.
>
> ◆ Pharmacological interventions should be offered only when psychological treatments have failed or are unavailable, as psychological interventions such as CBT demonstrate better adherence and outcomes.
>
> ◆ NICE guidelines recommend sertraline (SSRI) as a first-choice pharmacological treatment.
>
> ◆ In addition to sertraline, other SSRIs (escitalopram and paroxetine) and SNRIs (duloxetine and venlafaxine) are effective, as demonstrated in numerous meta-analyses and NICE guidelines.
>
> ◆ One meta-analysis demonstrated that duloxetine, followed by sertraline, produced the greatest response; escitalopram, followed by venlafaxine, the greatest remission; and sertraline, followed by pregabalin, the greatest tolerability.

Psychological treatments

The review completed for a NICE guideline on the management of GAD in adults, in addition to providing data on medication (as reported in the section "Pharmacological treatments") also reported on "high intensity psychological interventions," of which CBT was the most frequent modality. Twelve high-standard RCTs of CBT compared with wait-list controls showed an ES superiority of 0.63; eight of CBT versus applied relaxation showed comparable efficacy (ES = 0.01); and three RCTs that compared CBT with an active comparator showed superiority of CBT (ES = 0.59). It was concluded that the evidence base for CBT versus an inactive control is quite strong, and when compared against an active control, the evidence is less strong but adequate. CBT is to be preferred over medications because of the improved tolerability, although the cost per patient is likely to be greater. Despite the lack of statistically significant differences between CBT and applied relaxation on the majority of GAD outcomes, evidence supports CBT, given its larger magnitude of effect compared to applied relaxation (National Collaborating Center for Mental Health, 2011).

Siev and Chambless (2007) identified five studies that compared cognitive therapy with relaxation training and found no significant differences in outcome, consistent with the comparisons with applied relaxation. In a review of studies conducted from 1990 to 2004, Fisher (2006) reported that 34–37% of treatment completers who received applied relaxation interventions alone and 36–37% who received cognitive therapy alone achieved recovery at post-treatment (based on Penn State Worry Questionnaire [PSWQ] and State-Trait Anxiety Inventory-Trait Scale [STAI-T] scores), and recovery rates remained stable at one-year follow-up. Among individuals who were treated with combined cognitive and behavioral interventions, 46–48% achieved recovery at post-treatment and 53–63% at one-year follow-up.

Because of concern that few studies used worry, the core feature of GAD, as an outcome, Covin et al. (2008) analyzed eight studies that had used the PSWQ as the outcome measure. The mean ES superiority of CBT over the control group (any group that did not receive treatment or received non-directive or supportive therapies) was large (ES = 1.15), with gains being largely maintained at the 12-month follow-up. Hanrahan et al. (2013) extended the Covin et al. (2008) study, adding seven new studies that had been published in the intervening five years, many of which used newer forms of cognitive therapy (CT). Three broad forms of CT were examined, including treatments that focus on changing the content of cognitions (e.g., positive and negative beliefs about worry or cognitions related to uncertainty), mindfulness-based CT that aims to help people develop a more accepting relationship with cognitions, and treatments that combine CT with other approaches (e.g., motivational interviewing, interpersonal therapies, emotion-focused treatment). The ES superiority when compared with non-therapy controls was large (ES = 1.81), and when compared to active therapy controls (such as applied relaxation on its own), it was still 0.63, while comparisons with older forms of CT showed no significant differences. Gains were largely maintained at follow-up. The most recent meta-analysis, reported by Cuijpers et al. (2014), involved 41 studies and found comparable results.

Hunot et al. (2010) published a Cochrane Collaboration review of psychological therapies for GAD, with results that are similar to the NICE (2011) review. There were 13 studies of CBT compared to treatment as usual (e.g., supportive therapy) or wait-list control groups. The results of CBT were superior (RR [relative risk] = 0.64). Six studies compared CBT against an active control and there was such variability in the results that the difference (RR = 0.86) was not significant on measures of overall clinical response. However, there was a significant difference in the reduction of anxiety symptoms (as measured with the HAM-A and the Anxiety Disorders Interview Schedule), symptoms of worry and fear (as measured with the PSWQ and Fear Questionnaire), and symptoms of depression compared to supportive therapy, in favor of the CBT group.

Mayo-Wilson and Montgomery (2013) generated a Cochrane Collaboration review of media-delivered CBT and BT (self-help) for anxiety disorders in adults. There were nine studies of people with GAD in which CBT delivered by computer or book was compared with treatment as usual or wait-list controls. The superiority of the intervention group was ES = 1.02 and the results were stable at follow-up.

Internet-based cognitive behavior therapy

CBT delivered by computer over the internet (iCBT) is a rapidly growing field in respect to the internalizing disorders. Courses for major depressive disorder, panic disorder, and social phobia are common, while iCBT computerized courses for GAD, obsessive compulsive disorder (OCD), or post-traumatic stress disorder (PTSD) are less common. The first RCT of an iCBT course for depression was published in 2004 (Christensen et al., 2004) and, in respect to depression, the field is now sufficiently far advanced to have generated eight meta-analytic reviews, with that by Johansson and Andersson (2012) being the most recent.

The common model is a computerized course, delivered in about six lessons, that teaches control over emotions, thoughts, and behaviors using CBT principles. The results are straightforward. iCBT courses are more beneficial than wait-list control (Cohens d~1.0, NNT~2), and little sign of relapse is evident at six-month follow-up. iCBT for depression is comparable to face-to-face CBT in efficacy. Adherence in the research studies is high (~75%) and patient satisfaction is even higher. Adherence and degree of benefit is improved if there is continuing clinician contact (either face to face, by telephone, or by email) but the overall contact time required can be less than 60 minutes. As would be expected from the generalizability of CBT skills, comorbid conditions tend to improve along with the target disorder.

The development of iCBT for GAD is at an earlier stage, but the form of the courses and the results are similar. There are three RCTs of the benefits of an iCBT course specifically aimed at adults with GAD. Titov et al. (2009) used a six-lesson CBT course with weekly homework assignments compared to a wait-list control group. Robinson et al. (2010) used the same course over ten weeks and compared technician and clinician guidance to a wait-list control group, with three-month follow-up. Paxling et al. (2011) used an eight-week course of CBT plus applied relaxation compared to a wait-list control group, with a one-year follow-up. The results from the three studies were indistinguishable—there were 165 participants in all, and the mean pre–post ES on the PSWQ was 1.07 (range 0.98–1.14); the pre–follow-up ES was 1.33 (0.97–1.66), which was not indicative of relapse. The ES superiority of the iCBT group over the control group was 1.05 (range 0.96–1.11) at the end of treatment. This level of improvement is equivalent to an NNT = 2; that is, for every two people treated, one would get fully better (almost exactly comparable to the results of face-to-face CBT). Adherence (the number of patients who completed all lessons in a course) averaged 79% and the average time required by a clinician or technician, across the 165 participants, was 95 minutes per patient.

That iCBT for GAD is of benefit in research trials is one thing, but do such treatments work when the investigators depart? Mewton, Wong, and Andrews (2012) completed an effectiveness study of the program used by Titov et al. (2009) and Robinson et al. (2010) after it had been made available for primary care clinicians (physicians or psychologists) to use through http://www.thiswayupclinic.org. They studied the progress of 588 patients who were prescribed the course by their clinicians and had completed lesson one; 324 patients (55%) went on to complete all lessons. Non-completers tended to be younger and residents of rural Australia, but even the non-completers had demonstrated significant reductions in psychological distress before discontinuing. For those who completed the course, effect sizes on all outcome measures were medium to large, and over 60% of moderate to severe GAD patients met the criteria for remission at the end of treatment. Mewton, Wong, and Andrews (2012) concluded that iCBT for GAD is effective in generating positive, clinically significant outcomes in typical patients treated under the usual conditions in primary care.

The Clinical Research Unit for Anxiety and Depression, Sydney, Australia, which is where the authors of this book work, contains a specialist clinic that receives 400 new patient referrals per year. This used to mean that the staff could not keep up with the demand for CBT and that there was always a long waiting list. Long waiting lists are bad for patients and staff and produce malaise in the referring clinicians. It is now four years since we began to offer patients referred for face-to-face CBT for anxiety and depressive disorders, the option of iCBT. Nineteen out of twenty patients offered CBT elect to do iCBT at home. The cost of iCBT is much lower than face-to-face treatment, and adherence is above 70%, with benefits comparable to face-to-face CBT. We no longer have a waiting list, and referring clinicians and their patients are pleased. The clinicians now have time to spend with the complex and difficult-to-get-better patients, so they, too, are happy.

Transdiagnostic approach to treatment

Transdiagnostic treatments have been developed that target common pathology shared across mood and anxiety disorders. These treatments, whether delivered face to face or over the internet, are effective for individuals with GAD and are superior to control conditions (Erickson, 2003; Erickson, Janeck, and Tallman, 2007; Lumpkin et al., 2002; Newby et al., 2013, 2014; Norton and Philipp, 2008), produce similar rates of change across diagnostic groups (Farchione et al., 2012; Norton and Hope, 2002), and produce similar rates of change compared to methodologically similar diagnosis-specific treatment studies

(Hofmann and Smits, 2008; McEvoy and Nathan, 2007). Newby et al. (2013, 2014) developed an iCBT course for people with mixed depressive and anxiety disorders and showed significant changes on the GAD-7 measure, with ES superiority against wait-list control group of 0.85 (n = 99) in an efficacy trial and ES changes of 1.2 (n = 707) in an effectiveness study. Similar results have been reported in a comparison of transdiagnostic internet-based CBT (iCBT) to disorder-specific iCBT (Johnston et al., 2011; Titov et al., 2011).

Numerous transdiagnostic treatment protocols have been developed. In the first RCT of transdiagnostic treatment, Norton and Hope (2002) treated patients through 12 weekly, two-hour sessions that focused on psychoeducation, self-monitoring, cognitive restructuring, exposure to feared stimuli (*in vivo* or through role-played, imaginal, or interoceptive methods, depending on patients' needs), and reducing underlying perceptions of uncontrollability, unpredictability, and threat. This treatment protocol was superior to a wait-list condition, and 67% of patients no longer met diagnostic criteria following treatment. In the first study to compare a transdiagnostic approach to applied relaxation (AR) using the protocol already described, no significant differences between CBT and AR were reported, although AR had a greater dropout rate (Norton, 2012b).

The Unified Protocol is another transdiagnostic treatment for mood and anxiety disorders and consists of five core treatment modules designed to target key aspects of emotional processing and regulation of emotional experiences, including (a) increasing present-focused emotion awareness, (b) increasing cognitive flexibility, (c) identifying and preventing patterns of emotional avoidance and maladaptive emotion-driven behaviors, (d) increasing awareness and tolerance of emotion-related physical sensations, and (e) interoceptive and situation-based emotion-focused exposure (Barlow et al., 2011). These five modules are preceded by a module focused on enhancing motivation and readiness for change and treatment engagement, as well as an introductory module focused on psychoeducation about the nature of emotions and anxiety. The final module consists of reviewing progress and developing relapse prevention.

In a study comparing the Unified Protocol to a wait-list group, more than half of patients (diagnoses included GAD, panic disorder with agoraphobia, social anxiety disorder, and OCD) no longer met the diagnostic criteria for their principal diagnosis at post treatment (Farchione et al., 2012). Almost half of these patients no longer met the criteria for *any* diagnosis, post treatment, whereas all patients in the wait-list control group continued to meet diagnostic criteria, post treatment. Importantly, 64% of treated patients no longer met diagnostic criteria for any diagnosis at follow-up. There were also no differences in outcome across diagnostic groups, which is consistent with the majority of studies that have examined transdiagnostic interventions. One exception is a study demonstrating that while the treatment group improved more than the control group, only panic disorder improved significantly more than controls when diagnostic categories were examined separately (Erickson, Janeck, and Tallman, 2007).

Other therapeutic approaches

The majority of studies have compared CBT for GAD to non-active control conditions or active conditions such as AR or supportive therapies. Few studies, however, have compared CBT to other therapeutic approaches. Two studies have compared manualized short-term psychodynamic therapy to CBT for GAD and reported outcomes post treatment (Leichsenring et al., 2009) and at 12-month follow-up (Salzer et al., 2011). Both interventions led to significant, large, and stable improvements in symptoms of anxiety and depression. No significant differences were found on the primary outcome measure (anxiety symptoms measured by the HAM-A), although CBT was superior on measures of trait anxiety and worry, post treatment and at 12-month follow-up. Another study compared CBT to psychodynamic therapy delivered over the internet (Andersson et al., 2012). Both treatment conditions led to improved outcome compared to a wait-list control group, and there were no significant differences between the active treatment groups.

Research has also sought to examine the impact of enhancing CBT with adjunctive interventions. Integrating interpersonal, emotional-processing therapy to GAD may show promise for some

> Box 3.2 **Summary: psychological treatments for GAD (NNT = 2; NNH = 100+)**
>
> ◆ CBT is the treatment of choice for GAD. Research suggests that CBT demonstrates equivalent or superior outcomes compared to other forms of psychotherapy (both inactive and active control conditions) and to pharmacotherapy (due to increased tolerability).
>
> ◆ Internet-based automated CBT (iCBT) is efficacious (with benefits comparable to face-to-face CBT), cost-effective, and convenient.
>
> ◆ Transdiagnostic cognitive behavioral treatments (face-to-face or iCBT) that target common pathology across mood and anxiety disorders are also effective for GAD and address comorbidities.

individuals. One open trial found that this integrative approach led to significant decreases in GAD symptoms, post treatment and at one-year follow-up (Newman et al., 2008a). Effect sizes in the combined treatment group were greater than effect sizes of CBT reported in the extant literature. However, direct comparisons were not conducted in this study. In the first RCT, Newman et al. (2011) compared the efficacy of CBT plus interpersonal emotional processing to CBT plus supportive listening. Both treatments demonstrated very large effect sizes, with no significant differences between groups. Evidence also suggests that adding motivational interviewing techniques to CBT can enhance efficacy of treatment for GAD (Aviram and Westra, 2011) and anxiety disorders more generally (Westra, Arkowitz, and Dozois, 2009), compared to CBT interventions alone. Box 3.2 summarizes recommendations for the psychological treatment of GAD.

Questions for future research

What is the comparative efficacy of contemporary CBT programs and what is the long-term efficacy of different treatment protocols?

Studies need to examine the long-term efficacy of various treatments and should include a range of outcome variables, such as symptoms

(GAD-specific as well as symptoms frequently comorbid with GAD such as symptoms of depression), processes that are thought to cause and maintain GAD (e.g., experiential avoidance, intolerance of uncertainty, or meta-worry), disability, work productivity, healthcare utilization, costs, quality of life, and impact on families. There has only been one head-to-head comparison of contemporary treatment packages (CBT based on the Metacognitive Model and the Intolerance of Uncertainty Model; see van der Heiden, Muris, and van der Molen [2012]), and more comparisons are needed across various treatment approaches. Given that the components of treatment included in each model overlap substantially, mediation analyses are needed to determine which specific components of treatment are most effective.

Who does not improve following CBT?

We do not know a great deal about patients who do not sufficiently benefit from treatment. Although intriguing developments have been made with respect to the role of emotional processing and interpersonal difficulties (Borkovec et al., 2002; Newman and Llera, 2011), research is needed to systematically identify and describe the characteristics of this cohort. Such characteristics could include symptom profiles, developmental trajectories, and factors thought to perpetuate GAD (e.g., intolerance of uncertainty, experiential avoidance, meta-cognitive beliefs).

How does the "dose" and order of treatment components affect outcome?

At times, it appears clinically warranted to modify the order of treatment components from the order prescribed in standardized treatment protocols (van der Heiden, Muris, and van der Molen, 2012). The impact of this on treatment outcome is yet to be systematically investigated. Also, many clinicians work in settings where only a limited number of sessions can be offered. While optimal treatment programs are being developed, it is also important to examine the minimum number of sessions needed to achieve significant therapeutic change.

CHAPTER 4

Next steps for improving treatment effectiveness

Introduction

Pharmacotherapy, especially the selective serotonin reuptake inhibitors (SSRIs), is of benefit in generalized anxiety disorder (GAD) to the extent that it can be regarded as a first-line treatment for people who prefer medication to learning how to control their disorder. The two problems are tolerance of side-effects and relapse when the medication is ceased. Psychological therapies, especially cognitive behavior therapy (CBT), are of benefit in GAD to the extent that CBT can be regarded as a first-line treatment for people who prefer learning how to control their disorder. Adherence is high and the benefit appears to be long-lasting. What then are the problems?

Half the people with GAD remain symptomatic following treatment (Fisher and Durham, 1999; Hunot et al., 2007; Waters and Craske, 2005). While CBT is considered the "gold standard" treatment, it may be less effective in treating GAD compared to other anxiety disorders, although this does not appear to be the case with the internet versions of CBT. The basic or "traditional" characteristics of CBT for GAD include cognitive interventions focused on identifying and challenging negative thinking patterns, and behavioral interventions focused on exposures and relaxation procedures to target the physiological arousal associated with anxiety.

How can the treatment of GAD be improved? Cognitive and behavioral theoretical models of GAD have been refined, building upon basic elements of CBT and emphasizing different factors related to the etiology and core pathology of the disorder. Five models that have gained the most attention include the Avoidance Model of Worry and GAD, the Intolerance of Uncertainty Model, the Metacognitive Model, the Emotion Dysregulation Model, and the Acceptance-Based Model of GAD. These models have been reviewed by Behar et al. (2009) and Garfinkle and Behar (2012), and are summarized in the section "Contemporary models of generalized anxiety disorder."

Contemporary models of generalized anxiety disorder

Avoidance Model of Worry and GAD

The seminal work of Borkovec and colleagues saw the development of the Avoidance Model of Worry and GAD (AMW) (Borkovec, Alcaine, and Behar, 2004) which posits that worry is a way of avoiding emotional processing related to fear. Worry is thought to be a predominantly verbal/linguistic and thought-based activity (Behar and Borkovec, 2005; Borkovec and Inz, 1990) which can inhibit or replace the vivid mental imagery and consequent somatic and emotional responses associated with fear. The less distressing and less somatically activating verbal/linguistic activity may reduce anxiety and undesired distress in the short term. However, avoidance of emotional experiences prevents the individual from habituating and reducing anxiety in the long term (e.g., based on Foa and Kozak's (1986) emotional processing model). Treatment, therefore, includes exposure-based approaches to reduce avoidance of distressing affective states and situations. Relaxation and mindfulness-type exercises are also taught.

The AMW also posits that individuals with GAD believe that worry is helpful for problem solving and avoiding future negative outcomes. These positive beliefs about worry are confirmed and reinforced when feared outcomes do not occur. Cognitive restructuring focused on the belief that worry is helpful thus an important part of treatment, as is monitoring the actual (versus feared) outcome of worries.

Some studies have found support for the AMW. For example, individuals with GAD report greater fear of negative emotions such as anxiety and depression (Llera and Newman, 2010) and that "worry helps distract me from more emotional topics" (Borkovec and Roemer, 1995) compared to non-anxious controls. The findings of several studies are consistent with the theory that worry is associated with reduced somatic arousal (Borkovec and Hu, 1990; Lyonfields, Borkovec, and Thayer, 1995; Peasley-Miklus and Vrana, 2000; Thayer, Friedman, and Borkovec, 1996). Also, a recent study compared regional cerebral blood flow (rCBF) between GAD patients and non-anxious adult participants during states of rest, worry, and worry suppression (Andreescu et al., 2011). During states of worry, all participants demonstrated increased rCBF in temporo-occipital areas, and control subjects additionally demonstrated increased rCBF in the insula and amygdala (areas of the brain that are linked to emotional processing). The absence of activation among participants with GAD in the insula and amygdala is consistent with the AMW, suggesting that worry in GAD serves to suppress mental imagery and emotional processing.

However, in contrast to the theory that worry serves as a way of avoiding or dampening negative emotional experiences, there is substantial evidence to suggest that worry leads to increased physiological activation (Brosschot, Gerin, and Thayer, 2006; Stapinski, Abbott, and Rapee, 2010), as well as elevated ratings of negative emotion (Hofmann et al., 2005; Stapinski, Abbott, and Rapee, 2010), trait anxiety, state anxiety, and depression (Davey et al., 1992). Newman and Llera (2011), therefore, have proposed an alternative theory of experiential avoidance in GAD. The Contrast Avoidance Theory suggests that individuals with GAD attempt to avoid the experience of negative emotional contrasts (i.e., shifting from a positive state to a negative emotion). Indeed, some data suggest that the experience of a negative contrast is more distressing to individuals with GAD compared to non-anxious controls (Newman and Llera, 2011). According to the theory, worry is reinforced because it facilitates and maintains a negative emotional state of chronic distress and thus prevents the individual experiencing aversive emotional contrasts. This may help the person with GAD feel "prepared" for threats and reduce feelings of vulnerability, as well as reducing averseness when negative outcomes occur. As yet, there are no data to suggest whether avoidance of emotional contrasts is specific to GAD or common across a variety of disorders. It is also unknown if reducing such avoidance will reduce GAD symptoms. While specific treatment protocols based on this model have not been developed, new approaches may include exposure to emotional contrasts, such as relaxation techniques followed by negative emotional imagery to feared outcomes.

Intolerance of Uncertainty Model

Dugas and colleagues' model highlights intolerance of uncertainty (IU) as central to the development and maintenance of GAD (Dugas et al., 1998, 2005). This theory suggests that individuals with GAD find uncertain or ambiguous situations negative, stressful, and threatening. Worry may be seen as a method of reducing this aversive doubt and uncertainty. Avoidance and safety-seeking behaviors, such as reassurance seeking, procrastination, and excessive planning, are also viewed as ways to manage IU. Similar to other models, this theory suggests that individuals hold positive beliefs about worry. Therefore, individuals with GAD respond to uncertain situations with chronic worry given their beliefs that worry will either help them cope with feared events more effectively or prevent those events from occurring at all (Borkovec and Roemer, 1995).

The Intolerance of Uncertainty Model (IUM) also posits that individuals with GAD hold a set of beliefs that interfere with their ability to effectively address daily problems (Ladouceur et al., 1998). This "negative problem orientation" exacerbates worry and anxiety and includes beliefs associated with a lack of confidence in problem-solving abilities, perceiving problems as threats, becoming easily frustrated when dealing with a problem, and pessimism about the outcome of problem-solving efforts (Ladouceur et al., 1998). Dugas et al. (1998) also note that chronic worry leads to cognitive avoidance (i.e., strategies such as thought suppression and distraction to avoid arousal and threatening images associated with worry, as described in Borkovec's AMW). Thus, IUM-based treatment targets unhelpful beliefs about uncertainty, daily problems, and worry via a variety of cognitive and behavioral skills including cognitive challenging, behavioral experiments, problem-solving training, and cognitive/imaginal exposure. (For recent and detailed case illustrations see Chapter 5 and Robichaud, 2013.)

A significant body of research provides support for the IUM. IU is a more robust predictor of worry over other factors including positive meta-beliefs, negative problem orientation, cognitive avoidance, perfectionism, perceived control, and intolerance of ambiguity (Buhr and Dugas, 2006; Laugesen, Dugas, and Bukowski, 2003). The four proposed maintaining factors for GAD (IU, positive beliefs about worry, cognitive avoidance, and negative problem orientation) have been found to discriminate individuals with GAD from non-clinical participants, although IU most strongly differentiated the two groups (Dugas et al., 1998). Experimental studies have also demonstrated associations between IU and worry (Buhr and Dugas, 2009; Ladouceur, Talbot, and Dugas, 1997; Ladouceur, Gosselin, and Dugas, 2000; Rosen and Knäuper, 2009). Studies have found that changes in IU lead to decreases in worry, and that the reverse relationship was not found, suggesting that IU may underlie the development of GAD, and improvements in IU may be a key mediator for reducing worry (Dugas and Ladouceur, 2000; Goldman et al., 2007). There is also some evidence that IU is specific to GAD, not panic disorder with agoraphobia (De Jong-Meyer, Beck, and Riede, 2009; Robichaud and Dugas, 2005).

Numerous studies, however, suggest that IU contributes to the symptoms of many anxiety disorders and depression and may not reliably distinguish individuals with GAD from those diagnosed with other anxiety disorders (Boswell et al., 2013; Mahoney and McEvoy, 2012a, b, c; McEvoy and Mahoney, 2011, 2012; Robichaud and Dugas, 2005). A recent meta-analysis suggests that IU is not specific to GAD and is also evident in obsessive compulsive disorder (OCD) and depression (Gentes and Ruscio, 2011). Other research demonstrates that, in addition to GAD, IU is significantly associated with neuroticism and symptoms of social phobia, panic disorder and agoraphobia, OCD, and depression (McEvoy and Mahoney, 2012). Studies suggesting that IU is transdiagnostic have used larger sample sizes, which may have led to increased power to detect associations (McEvoy and Mahoney, 2012). Nevertheless, IU is likely to be highly relevant to our understanding GAD.

Metacognitive Model

The Metacognitive Model (MCM) (Wells, 2005a) explains that two types of worry exist in GAD. "Type 1 worry" refers to worry about external situations or physical symptoms. "Type 2 worry" refers to meta-worry and consists of one's negative beliefs about worry, such as the fear that worry is uncontrollable or inherently dangerous (i.e., "worry about worry") (Wells, 1995). According to the MCM, an individual's positive beliefs about worry (i.e., "If I worry, I will be prepared") lead to increased Type 1 worries, which then activate negative meta-beliefs. A worry cycle is maintained in which an individual interprets his or her worries as dangerous, leading to increased anxiety, which then leads to unhelpful strategies to avoid and control the feared consequences of worrying. For example, the individual may avoid situations that trigger worries, suppress thoughts that trigger worries, or engage in reassurance seeking. Such strategies are often ineffective and ultimately perpetuate anxiety by reinforcing the belief that worry is dangerous, as the individual never learns alternate coping strategies and does not have the opportunity to discover that worry is not harmful (Wells, 1999). Treatment based on the MCM rigorously targets meta-beliefs via cognitive restructuring, behavioral experimentation, and the practice of non-worry/alternate coping responses. (For recent and detailed case illustrations see Chapter 5 and Hjemdal et al., 2013.)

There is empirical support for the MCM. The association between Type 2 worry and pathological worry is significant and independent of Type 1 worry and trait anxiety (Wells and Carter, 1999). Both positive and negative beliefs about worry have been associated with worry and GAD symptoms, although only negative beliefs have been found to mediate the relationship between trait worrying and GAD symptoms (Hebert et al., 2014; Penney, Mazmanian, and Rudanycz, 2013). To some extent, Type 2 worry also appears to be able to distinguish GAD samples from non-GAD samples. Controlling for Type 1 worries, the *frequency* of Type 2 worry discriminated between individuals with GAD and those with somatic anxiety or no anxiety (Wells, 2005a). However, the extent to which Type 2 worries were believed only distinguished the GAD group from the non-anxious group, suggesting that elevated meta-belief conviction is not restricted to those with GAD. Wells and

Carter (2001) found that some negative beliefs about worry distinguished GAD patients from patients with social phobia and non-patient controls, but not patients with panic disorder. Furthermore, Ruscio and Borkovec (2004) found that select negative beliefs about worry distinguished high worriers with GAD from high worriers without GAD. However, the non-GAD high worriers still reported higher negative beliefs than a student sample, suggesting again that Type 2 worry may not be specific to GAD. Although positive beliefs about worry feature prominently in the MCM, the model does not assert that such beliefs are unique to GAD. Indeed, some data suggest that individuals with GAD do not substantially differ in their reported positive beliefs about worry compared to those without GAD (Davis and Valentiner, 2000).

Longitudinal and experimental research is needed to examine the causal role of metacognitive beliefs in the development of GAD symptoms. A recent study experimentally manipulated metacognitive beliefs among individuals with OCD and found evidence for a causal role (Myers and Wells, 2013), although no similar study has been conducted with GAD patients. Behar et al. (2009) also highlighted the paucity of research examining the causal relationships between Type 1 and Type 2 worries. Furthermore, no research has examined the relationship between Type 2 worry and ineffective coping strategies such as avoidance or excessive reassurance seeking. Head-to-head comparisons of treatment exclusively targeting Type 1 versus Type 2 worry is also needed. Notwithstanding these limitations, the MCM has greatly enhanced our understanding of GAD.

Emotion Dysregulation Model

Mennin's Emotion Dysregulation Model (EDM) consists of four central elements that perpetuate GAD (Mennin et al., 2002). The model posits that individuals with GAD:

(i) experience emotions, particularly negative ones, which are more intense than other peoples' (emotional hyperarousal);

(ii) have a poorer understanding of their emotions (i.e., describing and labeling their emotions and applying the useful information that emotions convey);

(iii) have more negative attitudes about emotions;

(iv) demonstrate maladaptive strategies for regulating and managing their emotions, which often escalates emotional states.

Consistent with the models already described, the EDM also suggests that worry serves as an ineffective strategy to cope with emotions and avoid uncomfortable emotional states.

Treatment based on this model involves learning skills to recognize, accept, experience, and regulate emotions in adaptive ways, and incorporates techniques associated with CBT and dialectical, mindfulness-based, and acceptance-based behavior therapies (for a recent and detailed case illustration see Fresco et al., 2013).

Some data provide support for the four elements of this model, indicating that individuals with GAD experience negative emotions more intensely, have difficulty identifying, describing, understanding, and regulating their emotions, exhibit increased fear of intense emotions, and engage in more emotional coping strategies (i.e., excessive worry, emotional outbursts, emotional suppression) compared to control subjects (Kerns et al., 2014; Mennin et al., 2005, 2007). Indeed, emotion regulation predicted the presence of GAD even after controlling for worry, anxiety, and depressive symptoms (Mennin et al., 2005).

Research is mixed, however, regarding the extent to which emotion dysregulation is specific to GAD compared to other forms of psychopathology. Mennin et al. (2007) found that various facets of emotion dysregulation were commonly associated with symptoms of GAD, depression, and social anxiety, although maladaptive emotion management and heightened emotion intensity demonstrated some specificity to GAD symptoms. The centrality of emotion dysregulation to borderline personality disorder is also noteworthy (Glenn and Klonsky, 2009). Other research has failed to support aspects of the EDM. For example, Decker et al. (2008) found that individuals with GAD did not differ from controls in their ability to discriminate among emotions, and Novick-Kline et al. (2005) reported that individuals with GAD demonstrated better emotional differentiation compared to controls. While previous studies have used self-report measures (Mennin et al., 2005), these two studies used different methodology (i.e., an observer-rated measure and diary cards). It is therefore possible that individuals with GAD give poorer self-reports related to their ability to differentiate emotions compared to their actual capabilities, and further investigation is needed. Additional empirical support for other elements of the model, such as the notion that individuals with GAD fail to use information that emotions convey, is also warranted (Behar et al., 2009). Furthermore, much of the research on this model utilizes student samples and more research involving clinical samples is needed. Most importantly, longitudinal or experimental studies are needed to demonstrate the causal relationship between emotion dysregulation and chronic, excessive worry.

Acceptance-based Model

The Acceptance-based Model (ABM) (Roemer and Orsillo, 2002) is founded on Hayes and colleagues' Model of Experiential Avoidance (Hayes et al., 1996) and Borkovec's AMW (Borkovec et al., 2004). According to the ABM, individuals with GAD negatively react to internal experiences (thoughts, feelings, or bodily sensations); for example, through judgment of emotional responses as extreme or undesirable and through meta-emotions such as "worry about worry" and "fear of fear." The individual is thought to then become "fused" with these transient negative reactions, believing that they are a defining characteristic of the self. Consequently, the individual avoids internal experiences believed to be threatening or negative ("experiential avoidance"). This can lead to "behavioral restriction" where the person with GAD avoids activities that are valuable or meaningful to them, either through engaging in activities less often or through being less present-focused during the activities.

Treatment involves education about the model and the function of emotions, mindfulness, and acceptance-based skills, and exercises to help patients engage in "valued actions" (i.e., do more things that they find personally important). (For a recent and detailed case illustration, see Hayes-Skelton, Orsillo, and Roemer, 2013.)

There is some empirical support for the ABM. For example, compared to non-clinical samples, individuals with GAD have reported deficits in emotion regulation and decreased levels of mindfulness (Roemer et al., 2009), greater levels of experiential avoidance and distress about emotions (Lee et al., 2010), and decreased engagement in valued actions (Michelson et al., 2011). Furthermore, restriction in valued actions was strongly associated with diminished quality of life after controlling for GAD severity, experiential avoidance, distress about emotions, and depression (Michelson et al., 2011). However, experiential avoidance is thought to be widely transdiagnostic (Hayes et al., 1996). It is unclear what ABM constructs, if any, are relatively specific to GAD, or if such specificity is important for treatment outcome. Substantially more research is needed to examine the model's components in clinical samples of GAD and other disorders. Longitudinal and experimental research is also needed to further evaluate the proposed temporal and causal relationships.

Comparison of the contemporary models

Each of the five models emphasize important constructs and have greatly expanded our knowledge of the disorder. The IUM and MCM emphasize cognitive processes, the ABM and EDM emphasize emotional/behavioral processes, and the AMW emphasizes both (Behar et al., 2009). Although expressed differently across models, each model conveys a shared emphasis on avoidance of internal experiences as central to GAD. For example, the AMW explains that worry serves as avoidance of emotion-laden stimuli such as vivid images and somatic activation, the IUM conceptualizes worry as a way of avoiding the distress and anxiety related to uncertainty, and the MCM notes that individuals with GAD attempt to avoid experiencing worry as a result of beliefs that it is harmful. Similarly, the ABM describes worry as a type of experiential avoidance of internal experiences, and the EDM explains that worry is a maladaptive strategy for avoiding emotions. Given that individuals with GAD seem to demonstrate an increased vulnerability for aversive internal experiences, it is not surprising that these individuals develop strategies to avoid such aversive experiences, fueling a vicious cycle.

Treatment approaches based on each of the five models overlap substantially, despite differences in the ways in which interventions may be labeled or described, reflecting the models' conceptual similarities. The aim of metacognitive therapy, for example, is not to reduce the amount of worry but, instead, to alter Type 2 worry (i.e., negative beliefs about worry), which is consistent with acceptance-based treatment, in which the focus is on one's reaction to thoughts/worries as opposed to attempting to change the content of the worry or reduce the amount of worry.

Treatments in all models include psychoeducation about GAD, the function of worry, and the role of avoidance. All treatments also involve self-monitoring of situations, thoughts, physiologic reactions, and behaviors relevant to their respective models. Arousal reduction skills are seen in treatment based on the AMW, EDM, and the ABM. All treatments also target one's relationship with thoughts and worries, such as through cognitive diffusion using acceptance-based treatment, belief reframing in treatment based on the EDM, and cognitive restructuring and worry outcome monitoring in the AMW, MCM, and IUM. Strategies to decrease avoidance and cope with internal experiences are provided in all treatments, using techniques such as exposure (e.g., ceasing safety behaviors, imaginal rehearsal, seeking uncertain situations, processing of core fears, exposure to threatening images or fears), or present-moment focus and awareness (through letting go of worry, mindfulness, and emotional/somatic awareness skills). Non-productive debates can develop when different terms or language are used to describe the same phenomena, which is critical to keep in mind when evaluating various models of treatment for GAD.

Effectiveness of treatment based on contemporary models

Approximately half the people with GAD remain symptomatic following traditional CBT (Andrews et al., 2010b; Waters and Craske, 2005). Randomized controlled trials (RCTs) suggest that treatments based on contemporary models of GAD are generally superior to traditional approaches. Table 4.1 summarizes these outcomes using intention-to-treat data when possible. Metacognitive therapy has resulted in up to 80% recovery rates, post treatment and at 12-month follow-up (Wells

Table 4.1 Outcomes of randomized controlled trials for treatments based on contemporary models of GAD

	RCT conditions	N[a]	Within group PSWQ post-treatment ES (Cohen's d)[b]	Post-treatment responder & high-end state functioning (%)	Post treatment, no longer meeting GAD diagnosis (%)	Follow-up outcomes
AMW						
Borkovec & Costello (1993)	CBT vs AR vs ND 14 sessions	55	CBT = 1.87 AR = 1.74 ND = 0.56 CBT = AR > ND	CBT = 26.3–57.9% AR = 44.4–72.2% ND = 16.7–22.2% CBT = AR > ND	—	6 & 12 months CBT & AR: gains maintained ND: some loss of gains; CBT highest end-state functioning
Newman et al. (2011)	CBT + IEP vs CBT + SL 14 sessions	83	CBT + IEP = 1.57 CBT + SL = 1.90 NS group differences	CBT + IEP = 64.7% CBT + SL = 58.3% NS group differences	CBT + IEP = 73.5% CBT + SL = 55.6% NS group differences	6, 12, & 24 months: gains maintained
MCM						
Wells et al. (2010)	MCT vs AR 8–12 sessions	20	MCT = 2.87 AR = 0.67 MCT > AR	MCT = 80% AR = 10% MCT > AR	MCT = 100% AR = 50% MCT > AR	6 & 12 months: gains maintained
van der Heiden et al. (2012)	MCT vs IUT vs DT Up to 14 sessions	126	MCT = 1.62 IUT = 1.08 DT = 0.03 MCT > IUT > DT	MCT = 59–80% IUT = 37–63% DT = 5–26% MCT & IUT > DT; some differences MCT > IUT	MCT = 64% IUT = 57% DT = 5% MCT = IUT	6 months: gains maintained

IUM

Ladouceur et al. (2000)	IUT vs DT 16 sessions	26	IUT = 2.13 DT = −0.68 IUT > DT	IUT = 62–65% (n = 26)	IUT = 77% (n = 26)	6 months: gains maintained

Ladouceur et al. (2000)	IUT vs DT 16 sessions	26	IUT = 2.13 DT = −0.68 IUT > DT	IUT = 62–65% (n = 26)	IUT = 77% (n = 26)	6 months: gains maintained
Dugas et al. (2003)	Group IUT vs DT 14 sessions	52	IUT (n = 25) = 1.23 IUT (n = 48) = 1.62 DT = 0.28 IUT > DT	IUT = 60–65% (n = 48)	IUT = 60% (n = 48)	6, 12, & 24 months: IUT gains maintained with some improvements evident
Dugas et al. (2010)	IUT vs AR vs DT 12 sessions	65	IUT = 1.16 AR = 0.85 DT = −0.15 IUT > DT IUT marginally > AR AR marginally > DT	—	IUT = 70% (n = 33) AR = 55% (n = 31) NS group differences	6, 12, & 24 months: IUT & AR gains maintained, only continued improvement evident in IUT

ABM

Roemer, Orsillo, & Salters-Pedneault (2008)	ABBT vs DT 16 sessions	31	ABBT = 1.33 DT = 0.63 AABT > DT	ABBT = 75% DT = 8.3% ABT > DT	ABBT = 76.9% DT = 16.7% AABT > DT	3 & 9 months: gains maintained
Hayes-Skelton Roemer, & Orsillo (2013)	ABBT vs AR 16 sessions	81	ABBT = 2.01[c] AR = 2.07[c] NS group differences	ABBT = 63.3–73.3%[c] AR = 60.6–78.8%[c] NS group differences	ABBT = 80%[c] AR = 69.7%[c] NS group differences	6 months: gains maintained

Table 4.1 Continued

	RCT conditions	N[a]	Within group PSWQ post-treatment ES (Cohen's d)[b]	Post-treatment responder & high-end state functioning (%)	Post treatment, no longer meeting GAD diagnosis (%)	Follow-up outcomes
EDM						
Mennin et al. (2012)	ERT vs MAC 20 sessions	60	ERT between group $d = 0.50–2.0$[d] ERT > MAC	—	—	9 months: gains maintained

Note: PSWQ = Penn State Worry Questionnaire; CBT = cognitive behavior therapy; AR = applied relaxation; ND = non-directive therapy; CBT + IEP = cognitive behavior therapy plus interpersonal and emotional processing therapy; CBT + SL = cognitive behavior therapy plus supportive listening; MCT = metacognitive therapy; IUT = intolerance of uncertainty therapy; DT = delayed treatment (wait list); ABBT = acceptance-based behavior therapy; ERT = emotion regulation therapy; MAC = modified attention control condition (i.e., supportive listening over telephone); NS = non-significant.

[a] All participants were diagnosed via structured diagnostic interviews (e.g., ADIS or SCID-I)

[b] Effect sizes (Cohen's d) were calculated using the following formula: (pre-treatment PSWQ mean – post-treatment PSWQ mean)/pooled PSWQ standard deviation; intention-to-treat data were used unless otherwise stated

[c] Statistics based on treatment completers (intention-to-treat data unavailable)

[d] Statistics reported by Mennin et al. (2012)—not computed by the current authors

et al., 2010; Wells and King, 2006). Intolerance of uncertainty therapy has been examined in group and individual formats, with up to 77% of patients no longer meeting the diagnostic criteria for GAD, post treatment and at follow-up (Ladouceur et al., 2000). Roemer, Orsillo, and Salters-Pedneault (2008) also found that 77% of patients undertaking acceptance-based behavior therapy no longer met the diagnostic criteria, post treatment and at follow-up. These findings are consistent with other reported outcomes (Hayes-Skelton, Roemer, and Orsillo, 2013; Roemer and Orsillo, 2007; Treanor et al., 2011). Preliminary treatment outcomes for therapy based on the EDM are also very promising (Mennin et al., 2012; Mennin and Fresco, 2011; Mennin, Fresco, and Aldao, 2012).

Only one study to date has directly compared contemporary models of treatment. van der Heiden, Muris, and van der Molen (2012) found that intolerance of uncertainty and metacognitive-based treatments were superior to a wait-list condition and led to significant decreases in GAD symptoms and comorbid complaints, as well as to clinically significant change, post treatment and at follow-up. The metacognitive therapy, however, produced larger effect sizes on most outcome measures, including cognitions related to both Type 2 worry and IU. Of note, this study did not examine the most recent version of the IU treatment, which has subsequently included uncertainty recognition and behavioral exposure.

More research is needed to compare treatment outcomes based on the contemporary theoretical models of treatment. Studies evaluating these treatments also need to be replicated outside of the research groups in which they were developed. Nevertheless, it is clear that such interventions have led to improvements in treatment outcomes for people with GAD.

Specific elements of treatment effectiveness

Treatment protocols combine numerous interventions. Mixing treatment components makes it difficult to identify which treatment components are most effective and should be optimized. To further improve effectiveness and facilitate the development of more parsimonious treatment packages, research has begun to deconstruct CBT programs to help identify active mechanisms of change.

Numerous studies have compared components of CBT (i.e., cognitive therapy alone, worry exposure alone, applied relaxation) and have generally reported equal effectiveness across various interventions. A meta-analysis of five studies compared cognitive therapy to applied relaxation and reported equivalent effects across all outcome measures, including anxiety, anxiety-related cognitions, depression, clinically significant change, and drop-out rates (Siev and Chambless, 2007). Applied relaxation has also been found to be equally as effective as worry exposure, in which patients were instructed to confront the image of their worst worry and experience the accompanying anxiety as intensely as possible until habituation occurred. Both treatments reduced symptoms of anxiety and depression at 6- and 12-month follow-up assessments (Hoyer et al., 2009).

No study to date has directly compared specific interventions unique to each theoretical model, with the exception of the van der Heiden, Muris, and van der Molen (2012) study, that directly compared metacognitive therapy to intolerance of uncertainty therapy. The active ingredients of these treatment protocols, however, were difficult to identify given the substantial overlap in intervention techniques across the two approaches and the absence of a formal mediation analysis. Therefore, the specific components of interventions that lead to change remain unclear, and more research is needed.

Mechanisms of change

Research suggests that specific symptoms do not need to be targeted explicitly for changes to occur. Such findings lead to questions regarding mechanisms of change and ways in which diverse intervention strategies might impact common underlying factors. In the van der Heiden, Muris, and van der Molen (2012) study, metacognitive therapy led to improvements on measures of IU, and vice versa, even though metacognitive therapy does not specifically target IU. Similarly, Treanor et al. (2011) reported that individuals undertaking acceptance-based CBT experienced improvements in a number of important variables including reduced difficulty in emotion regulation and distress about emotional responses, increased tolerance of uncertainty, and perceived control over anxiety. However, this study did not conduct a mediational analysis, which is necessary for determining the course of change. While the acceptance-based treatment led to changes in numerous variables, the relationships that may or may not exist between these changes and in the core symptoms of GAD remain unclear.

In the Hoyer et al. (2009) study comparing worry exposure (imaginal exposure of specific worries) to applied relaxation, treatments led to equal improvements in symptoms of anxiety and depression, as well as to cognitive variables such as negative metacognitions and thought suppression that were not directly targeted during treatment. In addition, secondary data analysis from this study found that worry exposure and applied relaxation reduced cognitive and behavioral avoidance, safety behaviors, and reassurance seeking, with no differential effects of treatment type (Beesdo-Baum et al., 2012).

A recent series of studies have examined symptom change in individuals receiving either CBT based on the IUM or applied relaxation (AR). Dugas, Francis, and Bouchard (2009) used a time-series analysis to assess the causal impact of changes in worry (targeted via IU) on somatic anxiety (targeted via AR), and vice versa. Results demonstrated that for most individuals receiving CBT, changes in worry did not uniquely predict changes in somatic anxiety, and for most individuals receiving AR, changes in somatic anxiety did not uniquely predict changes in worry. Instead, the majority of individuals demonstrated a bidirectional relationship in which change in worry and somatic anxiety equally predicted each other. The authors posit that changes in one symptom cluster may lead to changes in a second symptom cluster, which in turn impacts the first cluster of symptoms, generating a bidirectional relationship. Donegan and Dugas (2012) then conducted a mediation analysis to examine how GAD symptoms changed in relation to one another in a larger sample of individuals receiving CBT or AR. Results demonstrated that changes in worry occurred, in part, because of changes in somatic anxiety, and vice versa, although changes in worry were a stronger predictor of subsequent changes in somatic anxiety in the CBT condition. These findings suggest that different treatments may produce a similar degree of symptom change via different mechanisms.

Higher-level constructs that underlie various treatment approaches may explain improvements across symptoms in multiple domains. Based on their findings that applied relaxation and worry exposure led to changes in cognitions (which were specifically not targeted in treatment), Hoyer and colleagues (2009) suggest that both of these treatments may enable the patient to feel more competent when confronted with upcoming worries (i.e., through targeting skill mastery over somatic responses to anxiety in AR and by encouraging the patient to face anxiety and fears until habituation occurs in worry exposure). Both treatments may lead to increased self-efficacy and indirectly influence related negative beliefs about worrying. A shared emphasis on avoidance of emotional responses may also be a common underlying mechanism of action that all treatment approaches target. These theories, however, are speculations at this stage and warrant additional research.

The interaction between patient characteristics and treatment approach

Flexibility in utilizing treatment strategies based on specific patient characteristics and symptoms may be an important guide in choosing the most effective and appropriate intervention. To our knowledge, very few studies have examined the effect this may have on treatment outcome. In one study, participants' types of worry guided the treatment they received (Provencher, Dugas, and Ladouceur, 2004). Individuals were provided with 12 sessions of problem-solving training if their worries focused on current problems or 12 sessions of cognitive exposure treatment if their worries focused on hypothetical situations. Interventions led to clinically significant improvements in 74% of individuals who completed treatment. In addition, effect sizes for both conditions were large and similar to effect sizes obtained with the complete treatment package (Dugas et al., 2003; Ladouceur et al., 2000). The authors note that focusing on one specific technique may lead to better understanding and skill acquisition, and may improve treatment efficiency and reduce treatment costs.

Another study demonstrated that duration of illness moderated treatment outcome in GAD (Newman and Fisher, 2013). Individuals with longer illness duration responded better to more focused component treatment (i.e., receiving either cognitive therapy or self-control desensitization as opposed to the full CBT treatment package), whereas those with shorter duration responded better to the full CBT package. There is also some preliminary evidence to suggest that supplementing CBT with interpersonal emotional processing may be beneficial to GAD patients who report either a highly dismissive attachment style or a primary attachment relationship that is not enmeshed (Newman et al., 2008a, b). Adding interpersonal treatment to CBT, in select cases, is further supported by studies demonstrating that interpersonal difficulties are negatively associated with post-therapy and follow-up improvement following cognitive behavioral interventions (Borkovec et al., 2002), although some studies have failed to replicate such findings (Critchfield et al., 2007).

These results suggest that numerous unique patient factors, such as the types of worry, illness duration, and interpersonal and attachment histories, may be important in guiding clinical decisions about the type of treatment that might be most appropriate and effective for a particular patient.

Questions for future research

What are the mechanisms of change in different forms of CBT?

We know that numerous types of interventions are effective in reducing symptoms and impairment associated with GAD, but how do these interventions lead to change? Do various techniques act on different mechanisms or do these techniques impact common underlying mechanisms through different pathways? Answering these questions will help to guide more targeted treatment approaches and reduce redundancies within treatment programs.

Further research is needed to deconstruct treatment programs to compare efficacy across specific components of treatment. Time-series and mediation analyses have begun to examine mechanisms of change, and more research is needed using additive designs as a means of evaluating specific treatment components (Donegan and Dugas, 2012; Dugas et al.,

2009). Functional magnetic resonance imaging (fMRI) techniques may also help to elucidate the ways in which various interventions impact change in specific cognitive and emotional processes. While neuro-imaging studies exist for other anxiety disorders, no study to date has examined the impact of psychotherapy on individuals with GAD.

What CBT protocol to use with different GAD patients?

Clinicians need to know what theoretical model is best suited to different patients. Currently, this decision is based on the clinician's judgment, training experiences, and the patient's case conceptualization. Could the pre-treatment administration of pertinent self-report measures (e.g., measures of metacognition, intolerance of uncertainty, experiential avoidance) reliably guide the decision to provide a particular type of treatment? What other indicators could guide this decision?

Do contemporary CBT programs adequately address comorbid disorders?

GAD patients frequently experience comorbid disorders. The effectiveness of contemporary treatment protocols in addressing comorbid disorders needs to be examined and compared to the outcomes achieved by transdiagnostic treatments. A transdiagnostic approach appears to be at least as efficacious as "traditional" CBT for GAD. However, transdiagnostic treatments have the benefit of easier dissemination and improved outcomes for comorbid disorders.

How much training is required to reliably administer contemporary CBT for GAD?

Developments in therapy for GAD are continually evolving. Clinicians wanting to implement new treatment packages need guidance as to the level of training required to validly deliver new treatments. To answer this question, the effectiveness of treatment programs needs to be examined in naturalistic settings where degrees of clinical training and expertise are variable and the impact of additional training is evaluated.

Chapter 5

Clinical guides to treatment

Two treatment guides are provided in this chapter. The first is for physicians. It is brief, directive, and evidence-based. The second guide is for specialist clinicians who require a comprehensive manual for the assessment and management of patients within a cognitive behavior therapy approach.

Physicians' guide

Diagnosis is always the first step in treating any disorder. The core issue in worry disorder is to realize that although it is called generalized anxiety disorder (GAD), the issue is not generalized anxiety but months of worry over a changing range of possible adverse events that could occur, events such as illness or harm occurring to themselves or their loved ones. The worry is excessive and out of keeping with the threat posed by the adverse event, should it occur. Patients remain tense and aroused, restless and on edge, and complain of muscle tension. They avoid situations and activities in which the outcome is uncertain and could be deleterious. They repeatedly seek reassurance that the adverse event is unlikely to occur.

Physicians are trained to be good problem solvers and are happy to give wise advice. However, if the anticipated event is unlikely and worry is excessive, a sensible solution will provide no lasting benefit, and worse, having discovered how helpful the doctor is, patients will return with another concern. It is at this time that the physician should say "We've now tackled a number of your worries, do you think that you could be a worrier?" Most patients with GAD will agree, for excessive worry is part of their daily life, sometimes thought to be helpful but far too often experienced as exhausting and debilitating.

What to do? The steps in sequence are:

1. Direct the patient to a website like http://www.thiswayupclinic.org to read about worry and how to control it.

2. The patient could do the web-based, six-lesson, self-help course on controlling worry and sadness (because people who worry too much are prone to depression) at http://www.thiswayupclinic.org. Remember, the course will cost them (at the time of writing) AUD$55.

3. If that is not enough, you could prescribe cognitive behavior therapy (CBT):

   a) Guide the patient by using a copy of the "Patient treatment manual" in Chapter 6 of this book.

   b) Refer them to a clinical psychologist for face-to-face CBT (while using a copy of the "Patient treatment manual" in Chapter 6 as a therapy enhancer).

   c) Register at http://www.thiswayupclinic.org and prescribe the six-lesson course for GAD and guide the patient as they do the course.

4. If that is not enough, you could prescribe medication:

   a) A selective serotonin reuptake inhibitor (SSRI) in standard doses, but remember that the number needed to treat to benefit one will be five and the number needed to treat to harm one is probably about two. Sertraline is the best tolerated and among the most effective of the SSRIs.

   b) A serotonin and norepinephrine reuptake inhibitor (SNRI), bearing in mind that venlafaxine is often difficult to discontinue and can be toxic in overdose.

   c) Do not prescribe benzodiazepines or antipsychotic medication.

5. If the patient does not respond:

   a) Check the validity of the diagnosis of GAD and consider the salience of any comorbid mental disorders.

   b) If the diagnosis was correct, check that the patient complied with the treatments prescribed.

   c) If treatment was adhered to, consider getting a second opinion.

What a physician might say to a person with GAD

"We've agreed that you have generalized anxiety disorder, but it really is a term for people who worry too much over everyday things. You have been like this for a long time and the worry is wearing you down. So let us talk about treatment.

There are two treatments that work—medication with an antidepressant drug, and cognitive behavior therapy or CBT. They both work equally well, in that eight out of ten improve (five out of ten recover completely). Those on medication have to keep taking the meds to stay well; those who do CBT have to continue doing what they learned from CBT to stay well. CBT comes in two forms—seeing a clinical psychologist six times to start to learn how to recover, or doing a six-lesson internet course called iCBT at home, in your own time. Both forms of CBT are equally beneficial.

Thus, the three options are equally beneficial and you should say which you think would suit you best. The options do differ in terms of side-effects and out-of-pocket costs to you. Half the people taking medication report no side-effects; half have side-effects of which interference with sex life and withdrawal symptoms on stopping the meds are the most important. There are no side-effects from seeing a clinical psychologist for CBT or doing iCBT. The downside is that you have to discipline yourself to do it. In Australia, the out-of-pocket cost of face-to-face CBT is about twice the cost of meds for six sessions. iCBT is a third of the cost of meds. [The ratios between the costs to the patient of these treatments will differ between countries.]

Doing CBT and taking meds at the same time is slightly more beneficial than either treatment alone, so that's another option for you to consider. I would be happy to prescribe any of the options. Which way do you want to go?

Clinicians' guide

This clinicians' guide details a cognitive behavioral approach to clinical assessment, formulation, and treatment of patients who are experiencing GAD. Figure 5.1 provides a detailed outline of the contents of this guide. The (anonymized) case examples in this chapter have been

---

Assessment
- Clinical presentation—the signs and symptoms of GAD
- Differential diagnosis—GAD compared to non-pathological normal worry, other anxiety disorders, and depressive disorders
- Psychosocial context and history—assessing predisposing, precipitating, and perpetuating factors within a biopsychosocial approach
- Cognitive behavioral maintaining factors—assessing constructs indentified in current CBT models that are thought to perpetuate GAD (e.g., intolerance of uncertainty, metacognitive beliefs, cognitive and behavioral avoidance)
- Additional assessment considerations—patient goals, treatment context, comorbidities

---

Formulation
- The importance of formulation
- Metacognitive formulation
- Intolerance of uncertainty based formulation
- Avoidance-based formulation
- Alternative formulation models

Treatment
- Stage 1—psychoeducation, formulation, treatment rationale, symptom monitoring, factors that facilitate or hinder therapy
- Stage 2—CBT skills
  - o Addressing physical symptoms—arousal reduction and exercise
  - o Adressing cognitive symptoms—challenging unhelpful thinking about (i) everyday situations, (ii) uncertainty, (iii) problems, and (iv) worry (positive and negative metabeliefs)
  - o Addressing behavioral and avoidance-based symptoms—graded exposure, reducing safety behaviors and imaginal exposure
- Stage 3—relapse prevention

Figure 5.1 Contents of the clinicians' guide.

drawn from our clinical work, as have the numerous clinical mishaps and mistakes. The "Patient treatment manual" in Chapter 6 can be used in conjunction with this clinicians' guide and is based on our effective online cognitive behavior therapy program for GAD that is a routine part of treatment at the Anxiety Disorders Clinic, St Vincent's Hospital, Sydney (Mewton, Wong, and Andrews, 2012; Newby et al., 2013, 2014; Robinson et al., 2010; Titov et al., 2009).

Assessment

Assessment includes diagnosing and formulating the patient's core difficulties, as well as empathizing with the patient's distress, developing your therapeutic relationship, and fostering a shared language to describe the issues at hand. A good clinical assessment is therapeutic—for the patient and for the clinician! It brings structure and clarity to what can feel like chaos and confusion. Patients who experience GAD may present with an armada of complaints. Take Tom for example:

> "Doctor, I'm so stressed. I've been to see so many doctors; they tell me I'm OK, but I don't know, maybe something has been missed. I just have so much going on at the moment. I get so worked up; I'll probably have a heart attack . . . and work is crazy. It is so hard to get going and focus; what's the point? It's hopeless . . . my wife says I am too hard on myself, that I need to lighten up and stop thinking something bad is always going to happen . . . but I can't afford to relax. What if I made a mistake and my boss finds out? What if I get fired? We'd lose our home. My mother-in-law would make my life hell. I could be out on the streets . . . and then there's the wife. She'll leave me if I don't stop checking up on her . . . but what if she's cheating on me . . . some of the guys at the gym are so good looking . . . and these headaches are killing me . . . if only I could get a good night's sleep!"

Throughout this section, we will use Tom's experiences to explore the key components of the assessment of GAD.

Clinical presentation

People with GAD often present with general feelings of distress and complain of physical symptoms such as headaches, fatigue, insomnia, and gastric problems. It may not be apparent to them that their excessive worry and anxiety is problematic. However, repeated presentations will make this clearer to clinicians.

Patients with GAD experience extended periods of intense worry, the degree of which often fluctuates depending on psychosocial stressors. Patients with GAD worry excessively for months and years, rather than hours or days, and patients will often report that they have always been a worrier and sensitive by nature. Indeed, of all the anxiety disorders, GAD has a particularly trait-like quality (Rapee, 1991).

The worry in GAD involves chains of thoughts about the potentially negative consequences of future events. These chains of thoughts are difficult to control and typically involve lots of "what if [something bad] happens … ?" thoughts, which start as concerns about minor mishaps and end in disaster. That is, worriers habitually make the proverbial "mountain out of a mole hill." For example, running 10 minutes late for a meeting may lead to fears of losing one's job and becoming destitute; or accidentally ignoring someone in a social setting may render the worrier fearing permanent ostracism. Although the worry of people who are experiencing GAD is out of proportion to the actual contextual threat or danger, they worry about the same things that people who do not experience GAD worry about. The worry in GAD concerns everyday issues such as relationships, work, finances, safety, the future, health, politics, and world affairs. There are often themes or patterns in the worries including those associated with failure, perfectionism, excessive responsibility, vulnerability, and approval seeking. The excessive worry in GAD is distressing and is associated with a number of additional symptoms such as muscle tension, irritability, impaired concentration and sleep, feelings of being keyed up, and restlessness. These somatic symptoms are persistent and can trigger further worry, which can lead to the patient feeling that they worry "all the time" and about "everything."

Although, as yet, not part of the *Diagnostic and Statistical Manual for Mental Disorders* or the *International Classification of Diseases*, patients with GAD will frequently report using thought-control strategies, behavioral avoidance, and other safety-seeking behaviors to cope with their worry and anxiety (e.g., distraction, reassurance seeking, and excessive planning) (Beesdo-Baum et al., 2012). Behavioral symptoms are likely to be subtler than those of the other anxiety disorders because the patient's perceived threat may be more remote or amorphous. For example, a patient with panic disorder who fears having a heart attack when exercising may find it reasonably straightforward to avoid this seemingly imminent danger by ceasing any form of taxing exertion. However, the GAD patient who, amongst other things, fears dying of heart disease at some unknown stage in the future, may struggle to neutralize their fear by obvious avoidant behaviors. Instead, they may rely on a host of behaviors designed to reduce the probability of one day having heart disease or to reduce the distress associated with this possibility (e.g., by excessively seeking medical reassurance, adhering stringently to a healthy lifestyle, or avoiding television programs about heart disease). Additionally, patients with GAD demonstrate attentional biases. Compared to non-anxious people, patients experiencing GAD selectively attend to possible threats in the environment (Matthews and MacLeod, 1986) and tend to appraise ambiguous or uncertain situations as dangerous (Dugas et al., 2005). As such, GAD patients often report that they "always have something to worry about."

Differential diagnosis

Worry is the hallmark feature of GAD. Worrying is also normal. Therefore, the *first task for the clinician is to determine whether a patient's worry is pathological*. Some useful questions to ask the patient to determine whether their worry is pathological or subclinical are:

♦ How often do you worry? How much of the day do you spend worrying? On average, non-clinical populations worry about one hour per day, whereas people with GAD report about five hours per day (Dupuy et al., 2001).

♦ Do you find the worry difficult to control? People with GAD will often report that their worry is intrusive; it is hard to stop and comes into their minds when they want to concentrate on other things.

♦ How long have you worried like this? The worry in GAD is persistent; it is experienced for months and years, rather than hours or days.

♦ Has the worry significantly impacted the quality of your life? People with GAD feel their worry is distressing and disabling in some way (e.g., it is associated with muscle tension, impaired sleep, relationship difficulties, reduced work productivity).

♦ Did the onset of the worry coincide with taking medications or developing a medical condition? Clinicians need to discern if the worry is the sole product of a general medical condition (such as hyperthyroidism), drug use (including caffeine), or a withdrawal syndrome.

Worry is also experienced by people who meet diagnostic criteria for mental disorders other than GAD (Harvey et al., 2004). If the patient exhibits clinical levels of worry, *the second task for the clinician is to determine whether the worry is characteristic of GAD or another mental disorder*. It is realistic to expect that many GAD patients will report additional disorders of depression, anxiety, and substance use (Brown et al., 2001). Additional diagnoses are warranted if patients' symptoms are not better subsumed with the GAD diagnosis and if they independently cause significant distress and disability. *The third task for the clinician is therefore to determine the patient's primary diagnosis*. This can be achieved by considering which disorder is most distressing and debilitating for the patient.

In GAD, the quality or nature of the worry is the primary problem. The content of worries is less important than in other anxiety disorders because when one worry fades, another replaces it. The experience of excessive, uncontrollable worry about a host of everyday issues is what troubles the GAD patient. Patients may say things like "I always think something bad will happen—even if everything seems to be going OK. I just can't seem to stop worrying." Some patients do not have this level of insight and may assert that all their difficulties would disappear if a particular problem was solved. However, a careful examination of the patient's previous experiences often suggests that this is not the case.

Within DSM-5, differential diagnosis is informed by the focus of patients' anxiety. In other words, "what is the patient worried about?" Sanderson and Barlow (1990) found that the vast majority of GAD patients will report that they worry excessively about minor things and everyday life circumstances (specifically, family, finances, work, and personal illness). In this way, the focus of GAD worry is generalized rather than focused on a specific environmental trigger. If a patient's worry is limited to or heavily focused on a reasonably narrow set of concerns, other diagnoses may be more appropriate. For example, if the worry centers on fears of negative evaluation in social and performance situations, social phobia should be considered. Alternative diagnoses may be appropriate if the patient is morbidly preoccupied and impaired by worries associated with having a serious illness (illness anxiety disorder), being away from loved ones (separation anxiety disorder), panic attacks and their catastrophic consequences (e.g., losing control or dying, as in panic disorder), or weight and appearance (as in eating disorders and body dysmorphic disorder).

Like patients with obsessive compulsive disorder (OCD), GAD patients describe obsessional and ruminative tendencies. However, the worries in GAD are typically more ego-syntonic, self-initiated, transitory, and related to everyday events, whereas patients with OCD describe recurrent, unwanted, and ego-dystonic intrusions that tend to have a circumscribed and permanent focus (e.g., contamination, symmetry, or anti-social behavior) (American Psychiatric Association/APA, 2013). Moreover, the worry in GAD is predominantly verbal/linguistic (Borkovec and Inz, 1990), whereas obsessions in OCD may also involve images, impulses, and urges (APA, 2013).

The differential diagnosis of GAD and major depressive disorder (MDD) is complicated by the high degree of comorbidity and symptom similarity (Zbozinek et al., 2012). Patients with MDD and GAD often report low mood, although GAD patients are more likely to feel predominately anxious with low mood as a secondary feature, while depressed patients will report persistent low mood and anhedonia as primary difficulties. The only replicated difference between the repetitive negative thinking in GAD and MDD is the temporal orientation of cognitions. Worry in GAD is future-oriented (i.e., "what if ..."), whereas the rumination in depression is more past-oriented (i.e., "why" questions like "why did my marriage end?" or "why do I feel bad?") (Papageorgiou and Wells, 1999; Watkins, Moulds, and Mackintosh, 2005). Examining clusters of symptoms more specific to one diagnosis may also assist differential diagnosis; for example, muscle tension (GAD), anhedonia (MDD), appetite and weight changes (MDD), and preoccupation with guilt, worthlessness, and death (MDD).

The differential diagnosis of longstanding GAD and dysthymic disorder may be even more complex. GAD and dysthymic symptoms are similarly chronic, diffuse, and tend to fluctuate in intensity. Some commentators suggest that distinctions can be made between GAD and dysthymia on the basis of mood (predominately depressed versus anxious) (Shores et al., 1992), but others have failed to find reliable ways to differentiate between diagnoses (Rhebergen et al., 2014). As such, these distinctions may seem largely academic for the treating clinician.

Returning to Tom

Read Tom's initial complaints again. What diagnoses are you considering? GAD, illness anxiety disorder, major depression, panic disorder, OCD? All seem reasonable hypotheses given his symptoms.

The first task for the clinician is to determine whether a patient's worry is pathological.

Tom experienced multiple daily worries that were difficult to control. The worries concerned a variety of topics (e.g., his work, health, wife's fidelity, child's safety) and a host of associated symptoms (muscle tension, poor concentration and sleep, restlessness, and fatigue) that were distressing, disabling, and persistent. His symptoms typically fluctuated with life stresses but had gradually worsened over the last ten years, and had been particularly troubling for the last 4 years.

The second task for the clinician is to determine whether the worry is characteristic of GAD or another mental disorder.

Tom's worrying is characteristic of the cognitive and somatic symptoms of GAD. Although he sought excessive reassurance via medical tests, he did not attract an additional diagnosis of illness anxiety disorder because his preoccupation fluctuated and would often settle, with reassurance, for a few months at a time. Tom's fears about his wife's fidelity and associated checking behaviors could be conceptualized as separation anxiety disorder or OCD. Tom reported persistent worries about his wife having an affair when he was away from her and when he was alone. However, these worries were subsumed into the GAD diagnosis because his worries at these times involved multiple themes (not just separation) and included fears of being overwhelmed by the worry itself. Moreover, the diagnosis of OCD was not given because Tom did not experience these thoughts as particularly intrusive, ego-dystonic, or inappropriate, and his checking behavior was used to prevent his escalating worry rather than to neutralize a specific intrusive thought or image. Despite experiencing recurrent panic attacks, Tom did not attract a diagnosis of panic disorder. His attacks always occurred in the context of excessive worrying and, as such, were not uncued. Also, while Tom had worried that his anxiety would lead to a heart attack (or other catastrophic events), this concern was not specifically bound to his panic attacks.

The third task for the clinician is to determine the patient's primary diagnosis.

Tom's mood was primarily anxious, but he attracted the secondary diagnosis of dysthymia due to his prolonged and near-daily feelings of sadness, hopelessness, and reduced self-esteem for the past three years. Tom was most bothered by his worry and he felt that if he worried less, he would probably not feel as sad or hopeless. However, he failed to reach diagnostic criteria for a major depressive episode as he denied significant anhedonia, weight or appetite changes, psychomotor retardation or agitation, excessive guilt/ worthlessness, or recurrent suicidal ideation. See Box 5.1 for more assessment tips.

Box 5.1 **Assessment tips**

The assessment process affords clinicians time to genuinely listen to their patients' experiences, and to empathize and validate their distress. Many patients find it helpful to have their symptoms labeled as a diagnosis. Clinicians can use the opportunity to assure patients that the disorder is recognized and treatable, which can inspire confidence and hope for change. However, it is prudent to discuss what the diagnosis means to the patient and to address any concerns they have about it (e.g., some patients may see a diagnosis as evidence of personal failure, weakness, or impeding insanity; whereas others may feel relieved and validated to have a name for their difficulties). Including brief symptom measures like the GAD-7 (Spitzer, Kroenke, Williams, & Löwe, 2006) and the three item Penn State Worry Questionnaire (Berle et al., 2011) during your assessment can facilitate diagnosis and provide a quick but standardized way to assess changes across treatment.

Psychosocial context and history

In addition to diagnosing patients, clinicians need to assess current and past biopsychosocial features. This part of the assessment facilitates an appreciation of the predisposing, precipitating, and perpetuating factors that influence patients' presenting problems. Let us turn again to Tom.

Tom is a 35-year-old store manager. He is married to Zeesha and has a 3-year-old daughter, Abbey. He reported that he has always been sensitive and prone to worry. Tom is an only child and his description of his relationship with his mother suggests enmeshment, with Tom always being the "center of her world." However, he felt quite distant from his father. Tom described his mother as a very affectionate, but chaotic woman, who was easily upset and tended to clean and check things excessively. His father was also a worrier, but Tom believed that he managed it by working hard and drinking alcohol. Tom denied traumatic experiences, but recalled that as a child he was afraid of dogs, monsters, and being alone. He struggled to sleep in his own room for many years, but he made friends easily at school due to his friendly nature and sense of humor. He performed well academically and at sports—partly, he believes, due to perfectionistic tendencies. Tom never had difficulties entering into relationships, but struggled to maintain them as he reports becoming clingy, possessive, and dependent with girlfriends, fearing they will leave him. At age 20, his first serious girlfriend broke up with him, and he engaged in some stalking behavior until he sought support from the college counselor to control this (he has had no other treatment).

Tom met Zeesha in his early 20s and they married when Tom was 28. Tom's anxiety gradually worsened as his sense of financial, occupational, and family responsibility increased over the last ten years, culminating in the birth of Abbey. Tom enjoyed his family life very much. He described Zeesha as a sensible, independent, and capable woman, but not particularly warm and affectionate. At times, this fueled his worries about her fidelity, which greatly annoyed Zeesha because the worries were entirely unfounded. Tom's career was successful and the family were financially stable. He was physically healthy but tended to drink excessive amounts of coffee and energy drinks in his attempts to "stay on top of everything."

We can see that Tom is genetically predisposed to anxiety difficulties and has an anxious temperament. His parents' excessive worry may have contributed to his heightened perception of threat, and he has adopted some of the coping strategies that his parents modeled (e.g., worrying, keeping busy, working hard, excessive checking). Over the course of treatment, it became apparent that Tom held a number of underlying beliefs and rules such as "I am weak and vulnerable," "The world is full of dangers," "People will let me down," and "If I work hard enough and stay on top of everything, I can prevent bad things from happening." These beliefs are evident in his current relationships, and are likely to have been influenced by his early life experiences and relationships. Tom's current symptoms seem to have been precipitated by the birth of his daughter and the increased responsibility he feels for the safety and integrity of his family. His intake of caffeine may be contributing to his current hyper-arousal, in addition to a number of cognitive and behavioral maintaining factors.

Cognitive behavioral maintaining factors

Contemporary theoretical models of GAD (see Chapter 4) explain how various cognitive and behavioral components are thought to maintain GAD on a daily basis. These components include:

- triggering situations
- threat appraisals (i.e., worries and "what if ...' thoughts)
- beliefs about the self, others, the world, and the future
- metacognitive beliefs
- intolerance of uncertainty
- negative problem orientation
- experiential avoidance
- emotion dysregulation
- thought-control strategies
- behavioral avoidance and safety-seeking behaviors

One of the most straightforward ways to assess these factors is to ask the patient to recount recent worry bouts, one at a time, step by step, from trigger to resolution, until the clinician has a good idea of how the patient experiences the worry process. Common examples of the various cognitive and behavioral components are listed in the "Patient treatment manual" in Chapter 6, and may serve as a useful prompt when assessing patients. Clinicians may also consider administering self-report measures that tap these constructs, such as the Metacognitions Questionnaire (Wells and Cartwright-Hatton, 2004), Intolerance of Uncertainty Scale (Buhr and Dugas, 2002), Thought Control Questionnaire (Wells and Davies, 1994), Negative Problem Orientation Questionnaire (Robichaud and Dugas, 2005), Difficulties in Emotion Regulation Scale (Gratz and Roemer, 2004), and Acceptance and Action Questionnaire (Bond et al., 2011). These measures can identify specific problematic cognitions (e.g., the belief that "worry helps me solve problems") as well as indicate the comparative relevance of constructs. See Box 5.2 for further tips on assessing cognitive and behavioral maintaining factors.

Additional assessment considerations

A number of general considerations need to be taken into account during clinical assessments. Patients' goals, strengths, and motivations to

---

Box 5.2 **Tips on assessing cognitive and behavioral maintaining factors**

Assessing cognitive and behavioral maintaining factors gives the clinician the opportunity to introduce the patient to the cognitive behavioral model. For example, when patients describe key triggering situations, they can be encouraged to identify their worrisome thoughts and feelings. Patients can also be encouraged to reflect on the relationship between these factors and whether their thoughts and feelings change over time (e.g., "have you always thought this way?").

change can have an impact on the focus of treatment and indicate how well suited the patient is to CBT at a given point in time. Secondary gain issues may also be apparent; that is, some patients may be motivated to remain debilitated by their anxiety (e.g., for personal or financial benefit). Additional barriers to treatment also need to be addressed and can include factors such as cost, transportation, work and family commitments, as well as major life events (e.g., surgery, moving, having a child, legal proceedings) and how supportive the patient's social network is towards treatment.

The timing and context of CBT for GAD needs to be carefully considered when patients experience various comorbid difficulties such as serious suicidal ideation and intention, psychosis, bipolar disorder, neurodevelopmental disorders, and substance use disorders. These groups are typically excluded from research trials and, as such, it is unclear how effective CBT is for these patients. Problematic alcohol use or frequent use of sedative medications is likely to interfere with CBT for anxiety and will need to be comprehensively addressed before and/or during treatment.

GAD patients with comorbid anxiety and depressive disorders report more severe symptoms before treatment than those without comorbid conditions. However, they are just as likely to achieve therapeutic gains (Newman et al., 2010). Treating the primary GAD seems to result in significant reductions in symptoms of comorbid disorders (Borkovec, Abel, and Newman, 1995; Davis, Barlow, and Smith, 2010; Newman et al., 2010). One hypothesis is that treatment is addressing shared maintaining factors. However, it is sensible to treat comorbid disorders directly when they put the patient's safety at risk or are likely to significantly interfere with GAD treatment (e.g., comorbid major depression). It may be relatively straightforward to dedicate some therapy time to address symptoms of other disorders (e.g., behavioral activation for low mood, psychoeducation about intrusive thoughts, introceptive exposure for fear of anxiety symptoms) (for treatment guidelines see Andrews et al., 2003, 2013). However, the efficacy of doing so is unclear. GAD patients with comorbid personality disorders (most likely to be avoidant and obsessive compulsive) may have a poorer prognosis (Friborg et al.,

2013) which needs to be considered when discussing realistic expectations for treatment.

Formulation

> "The doctor pulled out this sheet of paper with all these boxes and arrows on it. We worked on it together for a while. It was me—completely me. I wanted to pin it to my shirt! No other doctor had ever taken the time to put it all together like that. I really felt that he cared and understood. I was relieved that I finally had a plan of how to manage this worry . . . and it actually made sense!" Tom

Patient formulation or case conceptualization is an essential component of clinical care. It evolves across therapy and is a collaborative effort between patient and clinician. There are a variety of valuable contemporary models for explaining the etiology and maintenance of GAD (see Chapter 4). We will present some sample formulations based on these models, and revisit the cases at various points in the "Treatment" section.

There is considerable conceptual overlap between theoretical GAD models. The empirical data, as yet, do not support the definitive adoption of one theoretical model over another. In short, there is no "one size fits all" for every GAD patient, and it is likely that most of the concepts and processes described in the models will resonate with most patients to some extent. Most GAD patients will report some degree of intolerance of uncertainty, metacognitive distortion, and emotional avoidance. Differences may arise, however, with respect to which processes are most relevant for individual patients. The pragmatic clinician needs to avoid seeing these models as mutually exclusive and competing, and instead aim to move flexibly between them in order to customize formulations to patient presentations and to promote richness and complexity in their case formulation skills.

Metacognitive formulation

This formulation of GAD is based on Wells' metacognitive model (1995, 1997), which is shown in Figure 5.2. This theoretical model emphasizes

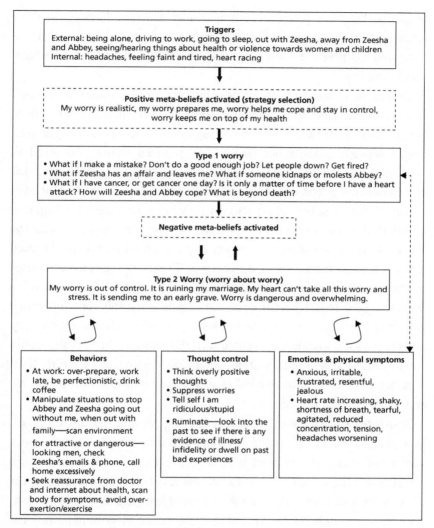

Figure 5.2 Metacognitive formulation of Tom's worry.

the role of positive and negative beliefs about worry, which are said to motivate and perpetuate excessive worry.

Tom's worst worry episodes occurred when he was least occupied (e.g., on his way to work or going to bed) and when he was away from Zeesha and Abbey. For Tom's health worries, there were internal triggers (e.g., feeling faint, tired, or his heart racing) and external triggers (e.g., watching TV programs about cancer or heart disease). In these situations, Tom perceived that something bad could happen and this activated his positive beliefs about worry. Worry became his habitual way of coping.

Tom contemplated a range of possible catastrophic outcomes (Type 1 worry), which led to distressing feelings that fueled more worry. Sometimes, Tom would stop worrying once he achieved a vague feeling or sense of reassurance that he had worried enough, "covered all the bases," or felt he could cope. This experience reinforced his positive beliefs about the value of worrying. However, with persistent worrying, Tom's negative beliefs about worry were activated. He began to worry that he was worrying (Type 2 worry). In an attempt to reduce the dangers Tom associated with worry (e.g., a ruined marriage), he used behavioral and thought-based strategies. These strategies were unhelpful because they perpetuated the GAD. For example, Tom avoided his worry triggers (e.g., by accompanying Zeesha when she went out) which prevented him practicing alternative coping strategies besides worry. This behavioral avoidance stopped him discovering that Zeesha would be faithful to him (Type 1 worry), and stopped him from learning if his worry was realistic (positive belief about worry) or if it would ruin his marriage (Type 2 worry).

Tom's reassurance seeking was overt (e.g., seeing his doctor excessively) and covert (e.g., asking Zeesha how her day was in order to check if she had come into contact with men), and was used to assure him that his worries were not true. Relief was short-lived, however, and the chronic reassurance seeking robbed Tom of learning that he could control his worry independently and that the worry was not harmful. The reassurance seeking also led to more worry triggers (e.g., frequent calls and insincere affection towards Zeesha led to arguments which fueled Tom's doubt about the stability of the marriage). Similarly, repeated body scans and doctor's visits ensured that Tom was very sensitive to benign internal sensations, which he subsequently misinterpreted as symptoms of illness due to his frequent internet research.

Tom also sought to control his thoughts. He pushed worries out of his mind by thought suppression and often substituted his worries with overly positive thoughts (e.g., "I'm not unwell at all, I could run a marathon right now"), self-criticisms (e.g., "You stupid man, you are so ridiculous for worrying like this"), or rumination (e.g., dwelling on previous relationship breakups or times of illness). These strategies exacerbated Tom's anxiety and low mood, and subsequently reinforced his negative beliefs about worry (i.e., "worry is uncontrollable and dangerous").

Lastly, Tom's emotional responses and their associated physical symptoms were, in themselves, distressing and anxiety-producing as they reinforced his fears that he was unwell (Type 1 worry), his marriage was in danger, and that his worry was harmful and out of control (Type 2 worry). However, as a way of coping with these aversive experiences, Tom again returned to worry.

Intolerance of uncertainty formulation

The next case formulation is based on the Intolerance of Uncertainty Model of GAD (Dugas et al., 1998, 2005), which is shown in Figure 5.3. Central to this theory is a specific cognitive bias, intolerance of uncertainty, which is thought to lead individuals to interpret uncertain situations as negative, unfair, and threatening (i.e., result in harmful outcomes), and to subsequently become distressed and avoidant in response. Jenny is another previous patient. Jenny had a variety of beliefs associated with intolerance of uncertainty, which influenced all aspects of her formulation.

Assessment and psychosocial history

Jenny is a 64-year-old woman who lives with her husband, Andrew, and adult son, Phillip, who has autism. She was diagnosed with GAD and MDD, and experienced occasional panic attacks. Andrew had recently recovered from a major depressive episode which developed during his transition to part-time work in preparation for retirement. Jenny and Andrew were reorganizing their finances which involved selling their current home.

Jenny experienced periods of major depression in the past, including an episode of post-natal depression when she had her first child, Mary. She battled with alcohol dependence in her early 20s, but with the help

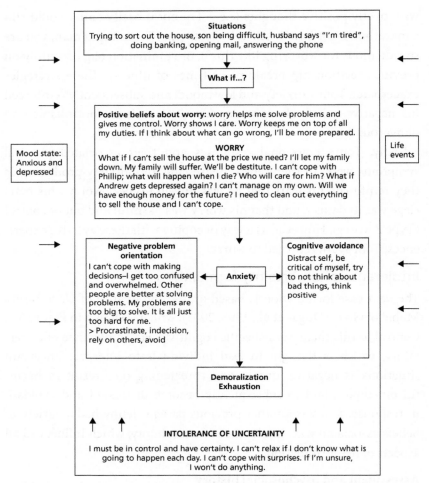

Figure 5.3 Intolerance of uncertainty formulation of Jenny's worry.

of her husband and counselor, overcame the addiction. In her late 40s, she developed breast cancer and responded well to treatment.

Formulation

Jenny's worry was triggered by a variety of situations associated with her and her family's well-being and future. These situations involved significant uncertainty and led to distressing speculations about future events (i.e., what ifs … ?). Jenny believed her worry was helpful in a number of ways and consequently engaged in prolonged periods of worry to help her cope. However, the worry (and the distressing images associated with it) led to anxiety and, consequently, Jenny engaged in a variety of cognitive avoidance strategies to cope (e.g., thought suppression and positive thinking). Jenny was particularly fond of distracting herself by watching TV with her son to avoid worrying about her finances and selling the house. However, this activity often triggered more doubts about the family's future.

Jenny described beliefs consistent with a negative problem orientation. These beliefs led to chronic procrastination and indecision, which prevented her from effectively resolving her daily sources of stress (e.g., returning phone calls, discarding clutter, and preparing the house for sale). Jenny's belief that she was not good at solving problems and making decisions led her to frequently consult others for advice (e.g., her accountant, daughter, husband, and physician). Conflicting advice and the increasing irritation and impatience of her advice givers further reinforced her belief that she was incapable of solving problems, which led to more uncertainty about her future welfare. The end product of this cyclical process was a deep sense of demoralization, helplessness, and exhaustion.

Avoidance-based formulation

We now turn to a formulation inspired by the Avoidance Model of Worry (AMW) (Borkovec, Alcaine, and Behar, 2004). As appropriate to our patient, we have integrated concepts from the Acceptance-based Model of GAD (Roemer and Orsillo, 2002) and the Emotion Dysregulation Model (Mennin et al., 2002). A central theme in these models is avoidance and unhelpful management of internal experiences (i.e., images, somatic sensations, and emotions). Worry is fundamentally seen as an avoidant process which is thought to inhibit or provide escape from distressing mental images, somatic arousal, and emotions. People with GAD may hold distorted beliefs about the helpfulness of worry and the harmfulness of internal experiences, which motivates the use of worry as a method of managing these experiences. However, it is thought that this avoidance precludes effective emotional processing which is needed for habituation and extinction. Thus, the worry perpetuates the intolerance of internal experiences.

Assessment and psychosocial history

Our patient for this formulation is Petra. She is a 22-year-old Masters student who was working part-time in graphic design while developing her textile installation art for an exhibition. She was dating Jillian and lived with two friends in a shared apartment. She was diagnosed with GAD, social phobia, panic disorder, and alcohol and substance misuse. In high school, she developed some symptoms of OCD (associated with germs and untidiness), but these symptoms are no longer a problem. Our visual representation of Petra's formulation is in Figure 5.4 and has been developed with reference to the figures presented in Behar et al. (2009).

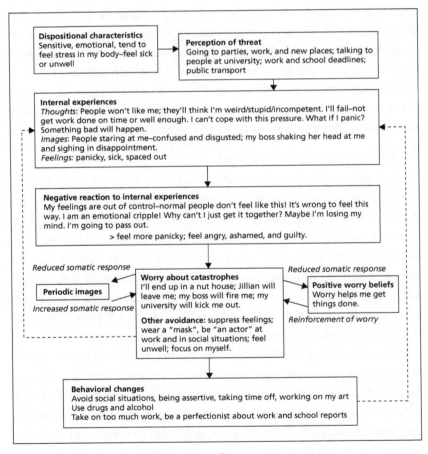

Figure 5.4 Avoidance-based formulation of Petra's worry.

Formulation

Petra had a sensitive temperament with a tendency to feel emotions more quickly and keenly than her peers and a longstanding tendency to somatize. External sources of threat triggered a variety of internal experiences (thoughts, images, feelings) for Petra. She responded negatively to these internal experiences with self-criticism and judgment which led to additional emotions such as shame and anger. To manage her increasing distress, Petra used worry and other avoidant coping strategies.

According to the AMW, worry is a verbal/linguistic thought-based activity that is thought to replace or inhibit distressing mental images and somatic arousal. However, during worry episodes, mental images return with their associated somatic and emotional arousal, and Petra again used worry to cope (feedback loop 1). This reduction in distress reinforced the use of worry as well as bolstering the positive beliefs Petra held about the utility of worry (e.g., "it motivates me to work hard and prepares me for disasters"—feedback loop 2). The usefulness of worry and the validity of these positive beliefs were further reinforced when Petra coped or when feared future events did not come to pass (e.g., "the worry got me through again").

Similar reinforcement contingencies operated when Petra engaged in other avoidant coping strategies which reduced her distress in the short term. However, some of these strategies, like suppressing her feelings, were cognitively demanding and increased the likelihood of negative consequences (e.g., Petra would sometimes lose the thread of conversations and contribute disjointed comments because of her self-focused attention in social situations). These experiences further reinforced her self-criticism and beliefs about the harmful nature of emotions. In the same vein, other avoidant strategies (e.g., somatization) directly increased aversive internal experiences.

Over time, Petra modified her behavior to avoid internal experiences (e.g., the use of substances, social withdrawal, procrastination, overwork, lack of assertiveness). These restrictions stopped her from doing the things she really valued and enjoyed (e.g., building her art portfolio and spending more time with Jillian). They also prevented Petra from learning to tolerate difficult internal experiences and examine the validity of her worries (e.g., discovering if her anxiety always goes on forever or if she needs to be perfect to be a good graphic artist) which perpetuated the cycle.

Alternative formulation models

There are several other formulation paradigms for clinicians to consider. Transdiagnositic conceptualizations and treatments address maintaining factors that are shared by the emotional disorders (Wilamowska et al., 2010). These approaches may be particularly useful for patients with high comorbidity or when providing group-based treatments (Norton, 2012a; Norton et al., 2013). We have found that simplified CBT models, such as the one presented in "Section 1" of the "Patient treatment manual" in Chapter 6, have been ideal when treating large (>100), heterogeneous groups of patients via the internet (Mewton, Wong, and Andrews, 2012). These simplified models may also be useful for patients who are working through a CBT-based program with limited clinical contact (e.g., bibliotherapy such as Lampe, 2004). See Box 5.3 for tips on formulation.

Box 5.3 **Formulation tips: mistakes we have made**

When we do not put a proper formulation together, our sessions are far more likely to be "figure it out on the day" affairs. We end up discussing whatever the patient presents with, which means that most of the time we focus on whatever has been upsetting that week rather than the important processes that maintain the GAD. Waller (2009) calls this "therapist drift" and we find that we do not get so off target in sessions if we have developed a good formulation with the patient at the start of treatment *and* if we look at it before every session.

Another common mistake we make is allowing our GAD patients to be over-inclusive or perfectionistic about formulations. For a decent working formulation, most of the time all we need is two or three typical examples of worry episodes.

Treatment

Treatments that involve multiple components, such as those proposed by Borkovec et al. (2002), Dugas et al. (2010), and Wells (1997), generally lead to better therapeutic outcomes compared to single-component treatments (e.g., applied relaxation or cognitive therapy) (Hanrahan et al., 2013; National Collaborating Center for Mental Health, 2011). Clinicians can introduce specific skills in the order prescribed in the "Patient treatment manual" in Chapter 6 or as indicated by the patient's formulation. For example, patients who spend many hours a day seeking reassurance may benefit from reducing these behaviors first in order to provide some relief from their anxious preoccupation. Other patients may be so somatically aroused that they require basic breathing and relaxation training before any other work can be attempted. The amount of therapy time given to each skill set will also depend on the patient's formulation and their response to interventions. However, as a guide, we have provided estimates of the number of sessions for various treatment components based on the literature.

Psychoeducation, formulation and treatment rationale, and symptom monitoring

Typically, treatment involves three main stages. In the *first stage of treatment*, patients learn about their symptoms and how treatment specifically intends to address them.

All evidenced-based treatment protocols of GAD involve psychoeducation. During psychoeducation, the clinician describes what GAD is and provides corrective information as needed (e.g., symptoms are not a sign of impending psychosis or dementia). Additional information about signs and symptoms of comorbid disorders is also important. "Section 1" of the "Patient treatment manual" in Chapter 6 provides information about the fight/flight response, and the prevalence, etiology, and treatment of GAD. See Box 5.4 for tips on psychoeducation.

Early in treatment, clinicians need to explain to their patients what treatment will involve and why. When developing a shared formulation, clinicians can guide their patients through their model using everyday examples that the patient provides and modify the model

> Box 5.4 **Psychoeducation therapy tips: mistakes we have made**
>
> As novice therapists, we tended to be anxious in our first few sessions with patients. We were still learning the psychoeducation that we were supposed to be teaching our patients, and our safety behavior was to talk too much and (most likely) confuse our patients with all the details. We forgot that anxiety inhibits learning and overestimated how much our patients could take in at once. Now, we make the education stage of treatment more interactive and ensure that our patients have something to take home with them so they can revise the material.

to suit the patient's experiences. Many patients confuse the difference between situations, thoughts, and feelings. So, avoid rushing this portion of therapy and instead continue with examples until the distinctions are clear.

Clinicians need to encourage patients to reflect on the relationships between the components in their model, and how the various symptoms reinforce each other to perpetuate GAD. For example, thoughts about "something bad" happening trigger the fight/flight response, which leads to urges to avoid. Avoidance can relieve anxiety in the short term, but it prevents disconfirmation of the initial fears of something bad happening and fosters beliefs that the patient cannot cope with facing their fears. The rationale for treatment then follows. Clinicians need to explain how treatment will systematically address the factors that maintain GAD (e.g., challenging beliefs that worry is helpful or learning to tolerate uncertainty and distress via graded exposure). Examples are provided in the "Patient treatment manual" in Chapter 6.

There are a number of therapy-interfering behaviors that are typically seen in anxiety disorders. These include avoidance (of therapy tasks and sessions), reassurance seeking, substance misuse (including sedative medications), passivity during therapy tasks, and dependence on the therapist. These behaviors need to be specifically included in the formulation and treatment rationale. The likelihood of rifts in the therapeutic relationship is reduced when clinicians clearly identify therapy-interfering behaviors and develop a plan for managing them at the outset of treatment. Reassurance seeking can be particularly problematic for GAD patients. From the start of treatment, patients need to be aware why clinicians will not provide reassurance (i.e., relief is short-lived; prevents disconfirmation of worries and meta-beliefs; fuels intolerance of uncertainty and intolerance of affect). When patients seek excessive reassurance, clinicians can suggest, for example, that the patient is doing so and remind them why reassurance will not be provided. A simple but kind reply like "I don't know," "I'm not sure," or best of all, "Let's wait and see" may also be appropriate.

Early in treatment, clinicians should also explain the nature and boundaries of therapy in general. It can be helpful to develop a contract with the patient that specifies expectations and responsibilities. Clinicians should consider discussing the following with their patients:

- The therapeutic relationship needs to be collaborative and respectful. Both clinician and patient need to trust each other and commit to maintaining confidentiality, honesty, clear communication, and safety (e.g., no threats or "surprise" tasks imposed on the patient or clinician).

- Treatment is an opportunity to be flexible and experiment with new ways of thinking and behaving. The clinician needs to be appropriately supportive, available, and knowledgeable, but the patient needs to take responsibility to try new approaches and avoid passivity or expecting the clinician to "cure" them. The aim of treatment is for the patient to learn new skills in order to become their "own therapist" and continue managing their worry, post treatment.

- Treatment sessions need to be regular (e.g., once a week), time-limited (e.g., 6–16 sessions is typical), and contingent upon outcome (e.g., every four sessions, progress is reviewed and additional sessions are contracted if the need is clearly evident).

- The content of sessions is present-focused and structured to systematically address the factors that maintain the patient's anxiety and to achieve the patient's goals.

◆ Homework tasks (for both patient and clinician) are essential. It may be useful to provide patients with a folder or exercise book to organize therapy materials.

◆ Guidelines on attendance and punctuality need to be explicit (e.g., therapy will cease if three sessions are missed; sessions will not be provided if the patient is more than 20 minutes late).

◆ There are many "ups and downs" in treatment. It is not realistic or helpful to expect that patients will feel better immediately and progress without setbacks, or that clinicians will have the "right" answer to every question or problem.

For more tips on setting boundaries in therapy sessions, see Box 5.5.

The first stage of treatment often involves patients engaging in some form of self-monitoring. Monitoring reinforces the therapy formulation and helps patients discover the connections and patterns in their symptoms. We have included a simple monitoring form in "Section 2" of the "Patient treatment manual" in Chapter 6, but it is likely that clinicians will include additional constructs pertinent to their patient's formulation (e.g., metacognitive beliefs and responses to them, or emotions and beliefs about them). Monitoring often involves patients learning to identify differing degrees of symptoms. For example, clinicians typically use subjective units of distress (SUDs) to gauge the strength of

---

Box 5.5 **Boundaries in sessions: mistakes we have made**

We often start a session with "How has your week been?" or "How are you doing?". However, with our GAD patients, this tends to encourage them to vent their worries or leads to a session chatting about topics not relevant to the problem formulation. We have learned that it is very important to set an agenda and structure sessions around the formulation, otherwise some patients come to expect a more supportive counseling session and can become quite upset when they do not get it. When our GAD patients really just need to vent, we agree to put a time limit on it!

different emotions (where 0 = no distress and 100 = maximum possible distress).

There are several additional options for intervention in the opening stages of therapy. The most common options are:

+ *Motivational interviewing*: patients who are highly ambivalent about treatment and the possibility of change may benefit from exploring the advantages and disadvantages of change.

+ Education for family members, spouses, or important others may also be warranted, especially if they play a key role in perpetuating the GAD.

+ *Bibliotherapy*: clinicians can suggest patients read pertinent books (or other materials) that will augment treatment sessions (a suggested list is given in "Section 8" of the "Patient treatment manual" in Chapter 6).

Cognitive and behavioral skills

After the first stage of treatment, we expect that our patients will have an adequate understanding of what GAD is and how it is maintained. In the *second stage of treatment*, patients learn multiple skills for managing their symptoms by addressing the factors that maintain them. For simplicity's sake, we have divided these skill sets according to the model used in the "Patient treatment manual" in Chapter 6. The section on managing physical symptoms includes relaxation training, breathing control, and exercise. The section on treating cognitive symptoms involves traditional cognitive therapy, as well as more recent approaches that address metacognition, intolerance of uncertainty, and negative problem orientation. The final section describes interventions that seek to undermine cognitive and behavioral avoidance, such as graded and imaginal exposure.

Addressing physical symptoms

Arousal reduction skills Relaxation and breathing training is used to reduce physiological arousal and consequently ameliorate symptoms of GAD (i.e., excessive worry). There is some, albeit limited, evidence supporting this proposed mechanism of change (Donegan and Dugas, 2012). Relaxation and breathing skills are not the mainstay of contemporary CBT programs. However, relaxation training has been employed as a stand-alone treatment (12–15 session programs) (Berstein and Borkovec, 1973; Ost, 1987). For example, Ost (1987) details an applied relaxation protocol which teaches patients to recognize the early signs of their anxiety and to systematically use their relaxation skills. Patients are first taught to progressively relax their muscles (taking 15–20 minutes), and then taught to relax in increasingly shorter durations (e.g., release-only relaxation taking 5–7 minutes and differential relaxation taking 60–90 seconds). Each form of relaxation is practiced several times a day for one to three weeks, or until the patient has mastered the respective skills. The relaxation protocol culminates in rapid relaxation (20–30 seconds) which is systematically applied in real-world settings that evoke anxiety. Patients are taught to frequently confront distressing situations and activities in order to deploy relaxation skills to cope with their anxiety. In their relaxation protocols, Borkovec and his colleagues (Borkovec and Costello, 1993; Borkovec et al., 2002) incorporate encouraging self-statements, relaxation imagery, present-focused attention, and view applied relaxation as an opportunity to extinguish anxiety. Relaxation programs are generally efficacious (Arntz, 2003; Borkovec and Costello, 1993; Dugas et al., 2010; Hoyer et al., 2009).

Relaxation techniques can also be taught as a component of CBT (typically 50% of treatment time) (Borkovec and Costello, 1993; Borkovec et al., 2002). "Section 3" of the "Patient treatment manual" in Chapter 6 provides an introductory rationale and procedure for arousal reduction skills as a component in a broader CBT program. For the pragmatic clinician, there are multiple applications of arousal reduction skills.

Tom: Progressive muscle relaxation helped Tom release tension and let go of worries before bed, which improved his sleep. It also became a useful exercise for Tom when experimenting with his metacognitive beliefs (e.g., "How effective is worry for solving my problems compared to relaxation or just getting on with my job?", "If I can focus on my relaxation exercise, how truly uncontrollable is my worry?").

Jenny: Controlled breathing was valuable for Jenny because it facilitated problem solving. Jenny frequently became overwhelmed by her problems and was tempted to procrastinate, but she used the controlled breathing skills to help her refocus and continue addressing problems rather than avoiding them.

Petra: Petra used relaxation and breathing training as a way to expose herself to feared bodily sensations and emotions. Arousal reduction skills were also used to help her challenge her beliefs that her feelings were out of control and that taking time off study and work was a selfish waste of time.

Exercise For global health benefits, the Centers for Disease Control and Prevention in North America recommend that adults aim for a minimum of 150 minutes of moderate-intensity aerobic activity (e.g., brisk walking) each week, in addition to muscle-strengthening activities for all major muscle groups on two or more days each week. Sessions of exercise need to be at least 10 minutes long. Multiple randomized controlled trials (RCTs) have found that exercise has a small to moderate positive effect on symptoms of depression (Rimer et al., 2012). It may also be helpful in managing anxiety symptoms and disorders (Asmundson et al., 2013).

Specifically in patients with GAD, Herring et al. (2012) conducted an RCT that compared resistance training, aerobic exercise, and wait-list control. Training involved two sessions of approximately 45 minutes, twice a week for six weeks, and led to significant reductions in worry compared to the wait-list. Remission rates were 60% for the resistance training (NNT = 3), 40% for aerobic exercise (NNT = 10), and 30% for the wait-list control. The authors concluded that exercise may be a low-risk and feasible adjunct to GAD treatment. Two additional RCTs involving small samples of GAD patients have also provided modest support for the benefits of exercise as a stand-alone intervention (Martinsen, Hoffart, and Solberg, 1989) and to augment CBT (Merom et al., 2008).

Box 5.6 **Addressing physical symptoms: mistakes we have made**

As with most interventions, adherence is a prime concern. Time and time again, our patients agree that they need to exercise or learn how to relax ... but do not. This is a frustrating and demoralizing situation, and we have fallen into the trap of advising patients just to "bite the bullet and do it" without properly exploring cognitive, motivational, and logistical barriers (e.g., beliefs such as "spending time on my health is selfish/wasteful/indulgent"). Dedicating time to overcoming barriers to exercise and relaxation has been particularly important for patients with high anxiety sensitivity, body image concerns, disabilities, and medical conditions.

See Box 5.6 for common therapeutic difficulties when addressing physical symptoms.

Addressing cognitive symptoms

Cognitive therapy Cognitive therapy is based on the premise that the way people appraise or think about events influences how they feel and what they do. The type of worries that characterize GAD typically involve overestimations of the probability and cost of negative things occurring, as well as underestimations of coping capacities, supports, and resources. This inflated perception of threat leads to excessive anxiety. Cognitive therapy instructs patients how to systematically evaluate the validity and helpfulness of worries through logical reasoning and behavioral experimentation. The aim of cognitive therapy is to develop more realistic and helpful thoughts and thereby reduce excessive anxiety.

Over time, themes or patterns may emerge in patients' worries. For example, a patient may describe a host of seemingly unrelated everyday worries such as "What if I can't do my job well?", "What if my relationship ends?", "What if others don't like me?", and "What if I make the wrong financial decisions?". The patient may engage in a number of safety behaviors to prevent negative outcomes (e.g., perfectionism at work, reassurance seeking in relationships, excessive attempts to please friends, and indecision in financial matters). Clinicians can explore relationships between worries and safety behaviors by examining the patient's most feared outcome if worries were to materialize (e.g., in this case, being alone and poor), and what this would mean to the patient (e.g., it may mean "I am worthless" or "I have no hope and no future"). Identifying and shifting underlying assumptions and core beliefs in the later stages of treatment may undermine a variety of daily worries.

Cognitive therapy has been effectively used as a stand-alone treatment (10–12 sessions) (Arntz, 2003; Butler et al., 1991) and as a component of CBT programs (around 50% of therapy time) (Borkovec et al., 2002; Robinson et al., 2010). Our "Patient treatment manual" in Chapter 6 provides a cognitive therapy rationale and examples of cognitive challenging and behavioral experiments (see "Section 4"). A comprehensive discussion about treating underlying assumptions and core beliefs is beyond the scope of this chapter, but interested readers may begin by considering Mooney and Padesky (2000) and Padesky (1994).

See Boxes 5.7 and 5.8 for therapeutic tips and common difficulties during cognitive therapy.

Tom: Cognitive therapy helped Tom challenge his worries that he would get fired if he made mistakes. Tom's perfectionistic checking prevented him from discovering the true probability and cost of making mistakes, so a series of behavioral experiments explored the real outcomes of purposefully making everyday mistakes and delegating tasks to others. Cognitive therapy also challenged Tom's underlying belief that as long as he worked hard and stayed on top of everything, he could prevent bad things from happening. Tom experimented with reducing his workload and caffeine intake and examined if any negative consequences occurred.

Petra: Cognitive restructuring and behavioral experiments targeted Petra's fears of failing and being judged by others, as well as her worries about fainting and losing control during her panic

Box 5.7 **Cognitive therapy tips**

Some patients may struggle to identify specific worries and instead relay general feelings, physical sensations, or beliefs about not coping (e.g., "I don't think anything, I just feel really frightened and shaky, like I can't deal with the situation"). It helps to validate these experiences and then assist the patient to uncover more concrete worries.

Ideally, clinicians need to refine worries until they are observable, measurable predictions about a specific "something bad" occurring at a nominated point in time. Often, it helps to use the "downward arrow technique" which involves repeatedly asking the patient "What is the worst that could happen here?" and "If that were to happen, what would be the worst things about that?". Imagery can also facilitate worry identification and shape vague concerns into observable behaviors (e.g., asking the patient "If I was making a movie of the absolute worst case scenario coming true, what would I actually see in the film?" or "If I were to take a photo of you 'not coping' what would it look like?"). Clues can also be found by examining the patient's action urges (e.g., patients may say "I don't know what I'm worried about, but I just know I need to phone home/take a tablet/wash my hands") and what could happen if those actions were inhibited. Monitoring thoughts during exposure exercises may also clarify specific fears.

If specific worries cannot be identified, clinicians still need to ensure that predictions are measurable and testable (e.g., the thought "I will be overwhelmed" could be refined to "I will feel anxiety 100/100, shame 70/100, and disgust 50/100 for 12 hours straight").

attacks. Introceptive exposure-based behavioral experiments were also used to test how uncontrollable and dangerous Petra's feelings were generally. Moreover, cognitive therapy was used to challenge Petra's beliefs that her emotions were wrong, self-indulgent, and abnormal. Behavioral experiments involved surveying people about their experiences of various emotions

Box 5.8 Cognitive therapy: mistakes we have made

The "rational" thought can seem so obvious to clinicians. Although we are well-meaning, we can fall into arguing with our patients and trying to convince them of the "right" way to think. Patients resist this, often passively by agreeing with us and then not changing their behavior. Therapists and patients end up feeling defeated and frustrated. Cognitive therapy works best when we do not assume responsibility for "changing" our patients' thoughts, but instead encourage them to be more flexible and curious in their thinking by considering alternatives. Padesky's (1993) suggestions on guided discovery are invaluable. More often than not, thought challenging does not seem real or believable to patients until they conduct behavioral experiments and complete exposure exercises. We have learned to accept that cognitive change takes time and worries are often related to deeply held beliefs.

Sometimes, cognitive therapy feels like we are avoiding uncomfortable thoughts and feelings (for both therapist and the patient). Good cognitive therapy is not about providing excessive reassurance, promoting perfectionism, or eradicating uncertainty and distress. We should notice when our desires to feel competent and in control lead us to "have all the answers" for our patients. This has been particularly unhelpful for our patients who struggle with feelings of inadequacy and vulnerability. The more cognitive therapy we have done, the more comfortable we have become with silences and reflecting questions back to patients (e.g., saying something like "Good question. I'm not sure. What do you think given your experiences and the work we have been doing?"). It often does not feel comfortable (for the patient or us!) to delve into the meaning, feelings, and images associated with our patients' worries, but cognitive work is more satisfying and effective when patients' emotions are activated in the therapy room.

in social situations and when deadlines were looming. This encouraged Petra to see that although she felt her emotions more strongly than other people, her feelings were not abnormal or depraved. Experiments involving discussions with her partner and boss about the role of emotions in relationships and work helped Petra generate alternate viewpoints such as "my emotions make me more creative, caring, empathetic, and expressive."

Intolerance of uncertainty Intolerance of uncertainty (IU) is a cognitive bias whereby uncertain situations are seen as essentially dangerous and unfair and, as such, are anxiety-provoking and avoided. IU is thought to drive excessive worry and, therefore, is a primary target for treatment (Dugas et al., 2010). Therapy targets IU directly via cognitive restructuring and behavioral exposure, typically over three sessions, as well as indirectly when other treatment components are delivered (e.g., problem-orientation training and cognitive exposure). The aim of IU therapy is to help patients discover that they can cope with uncertainty and that, for the most part, it is unavoidable. Therapy also aims to cease behavioral manifestations of IU such as excessive checking, reassurance seeking, and avoiding uncertain situations. Some practical guidance on reducing patients' IU is provided in "Section 4" of the "Patient treatment manual" in Chapter 6.

Jenny: During therapy, Jenny examined the evidence that she could not cope with situations where she was unsure and not in complete control. She recalled her experiences with postnatal depression, alcohol dependence, and breast cancer, and concluded that she actually did have the capacity to deal with very difficult situations that involved a lot of uncertainty. Jenny came to understand that although her son's autism meant that he needed a very predictable and structured daily routine, she had used this structure to avoid her own anxieties about uncertainty. Jenny devised a variety of behavioral experiments around reducing her reassurance seeking and being spontaneous and unplanned. She decided what to do for fun by the roll of a dice, she caught a train without knowing where it would go, and she tried new restaurants. Not only did Jenny find that she could cope with uncertainty, but she found the tasks were liberating and enjoyable.

Negative problem orientation Patients with GAD understand what to do to solve their problems, but their negative beliefs about their problems and their problem-solving capacity inhibit their ability to address daily problems. This is called "negative problem orientation" (Ladouceur et al., 1998). In therapy based on the IU model, patients are taught problem-orientation skills. The number of sessions used to do this varies across treatment protocols; three sessions in Dugas et al. (2010), seven sessions in Provencher, Dugas, and Ladouceur (2004), and four sessions in van der Heiden, Muris, and van der Molen (2012). Initial sessions help patients understand the difference between problems that are amenable to problem solving and those that are not. Patients are taught to ask themselves firstly "Is there strong evidence that this problem already exists (or is imminent)?" and, secondly, "Can I do anything about this problem?". If the answer is clearly yes to both questions, then problem solving is indicated.

Typical current problems are given in "Section 4" of the "Patient treatment manual" in Chapter 6 and are generally associated with a host of avoidant behaviors (e.g., procrastination, passive communication, perfectionism, reassurance seeking) that reinforce beliefs that problems are threatening and unsolvable. Hypothetical problems that may or may not occur at some unknown point in the future are generally not addressed by problem solving.

A structured problem-solving technique is outlined in "Section 4" of the "Patient treatment manual" in Chapter 6 (based on Andrews et al., 2003). However, as patients do not have problem-solving deficits per se, the bulk of the work for clinicians is to challenge patients' negative beliefs about problems. Once this is well underway, implementing the structured problem-solving technique will be more straightforward. Cognitive restructuring may help erode beliefs that problems are sources of overwhelming threat beyond patients' coping capacity (e.g., examining the evidence that "my problems are insurmountable" or "I am no good at solving problems"). Provencher, Dugas, and Ladouceur (2004,

p. 408) suggest that clinicians need to help patients consider alternative views such as "problems are a normal part of life" or "problems are challenges to be met rather than threats to be avoided." Robichaud (2013) suggests presenting problems along a continuum of 100% threatening to 100% opportunity-laden, and encouraging the patient to consider the potential benefits and opportunities within problems.

Obviously, the ideal behavioral experiment is to solve a problem using the structured problem-solving technique and then to compare the outcome of this process to the outcome that was predicted (e.g., "I'll never find a solution—this problem is too big for me").

See Boxes 5.9 and 5.10 for therapy tips and common difficulties with problem solving.

Jenny: Jenny used problem-orientation training to help her manage worries about her finances and moving. She understood the problem-solving method, but became easily overwhelmed by thoughts about the size of the problem and her inability to cope (her family had lived there for over 20 years and the house was quite cluttered). The problem-solving technique helped Jenny to avoid procrastinating and abdicating decision making to others. Instead, we worked to break the problem down into manageable pieces (e.g., selling/ discarding furniture, helping her son cope with the thought of moving, developing

---

Box 5.9 Tolerating uncertainty and solving problems: therapy tips

Dugas and Ladouceur (2000) note that GAD patients often struggle with ambiguous or uncertain elements of problems and the problem-solving process. Clinicians need to encourage patients to tolerate this uncertainty by, for example, beginning to solve problems even though the outcome is unclear, and by staying focused on the core components of the problem and avoiding getting sidetracked by minor details. These authors argue that a compromise needs to be made between avoiding the problem situation and gathering excessive amounts of information.

Box 5.10 **Solving problems: mistakes we have made**

Our GAD patients often arrive to sessions with a problem or crisis that is worrying them. It is not uncommon for us to spend the majority of the session coming up with solutions, only to find at the next session that our "excellent advice" has not been followed and there is a new crisis to address. Sound familiar? In hindsight, we can see how we have been drawn into the drama of the crisis and acted to relieve the immediate anxiety (ours and the patient's!) rather than systematically working to erode the patient's negative problem orientation and to build their self-efficacy.

---

a budget with Andrew). Although Jenny employed some gardeners, cleaners, and movers to help her, we viewed this as adaptive rather than another unhelpful instance of relying on others to cope. Interestingly, the house was sold during the follow-up period of treatment, which provided excellent evidence to refute her worries.

Metacognition The Metacognitive Model of GAD (Wells, 1999) proposes that excessive worry is maintained by beliefs that worry is paradoxically positive and negative, beneficial and dangerous. There is evidence to suggest that metacognitive therapy is the most efficacious stand-alone treatment for GAD (typically 8–14 sessions) (van der Heiden, Muris, and van der Molen, 2012; Wells et al., 2010). Challenging positive beliefs about worry is also a specific component of IU therapy: one session in Dugas et al. (2010) and Provencher et al. (2004); and five sessions in van der Heiden, Muris, and van der Molen (2012).

Metacognitive therapy aims to systematically modify unhelpful beliefs about worry via cognitive challenging, behavioral experimentation, and the cessation of thought- control strategies and other avoidant behaviors. Metacognitive therapy does not address the content of worry (as in cognitive therapy) but, rather, the beliefs purported to drive the process of worry. It is not uncommon for GAD patients to respond positively when the content of their worries is well challenged (e.g., discovering that, contrary to expectations, one will not be fired for making a minor mistake at work). However, on many occasions, a new worry will arise to take the place of the old one, and cognitive therapy tasks will need to be repeated. Metacognitive therapy aims to undermine this process by eroding the beliefs that perpetuate the use of worry, regardless of the situation associated with the anxiety. Wells (1999) recommends addressing beliefs about the uncontrollability of patients' worry first, then modifying beliefs about the dangers of worrying, before challenging positive meta-beliefs and eliminating cognitive and behavioral avoidance. "Section 5" of the "Patient treatment manual" in Chapter 6 provides guidelines for these skills.

Tom: Tom challenged his belief that his worry was uncontrollable by purposefully worrying for given periods of time. He did this with and without the therapist, and with and without added introceptive exposure in order to target fears of having a heart attack and not coping when alone. He found scheduled worry time (see "Imaginal exposure" in the section "Addressing behavioral and avoidance-based symptoms") and progressive muscle relaxation useful to reinforce that he did actually have some control over his worrying.

Tom also examined the evidence for and against his belief that his worry was ruining his marriage. Over time, Tom concluded that his worry was not destroying his relationship because Zeesha could not read his mind. The real problem in the relationship, for Zeesha, were his intrusive checking behaviors. These checking behaviors were slowly reduced and Tom also worked to limit his cognitive avoidance, notably his self-criticism and rumination concerning previous bad relationships. As an alternative to worry and checking, Tom spent more quality time with Zeesha and helped her around the house. As his depression reduced and the quality time increased, Tom and Zeesha were able to rekindle their sex life, which further eroded Tom's beliefs that his worry was ruining the marriage.

We also challenged positive meta-beliefs specific to Tom's worries, which included "My worry helps me stay on top of my health." Tom weighed up the various factors that keep people healthy. On the one hand, he could worry about getting terminally ill, or he could eat healthily, exercise regularly, limit his intake of alcohol, and follow his physician's recommendations. Tom saw that, if anything, his worry actually made it less likely that he would engage in health-promoting behaviors, and that his excessive reassurance seeking (e.g., doctor's visits, internet research, monitoring bodily symptoms) was giving him the false impression that he was looking after his health. Dropping these checking behaviors and engaging in regular exercise also helped improve Tom's mood and energy levels.

Letting go of worry Metacognitive therapy involves patients developing alternatives to worrying when a trigger thought comes into their mind or when they are confronted with threatening situations. One option is to generate possible positive outcomes to "what if ...?" thoughts (Wells, 1999). However "detached mindfulness" is viewed as the ideal (non) response (Wells, 2005b). Patients need to learn to let trigger thoughts come and go without engaging with them via worry or reassurance seeking, for example. The idea is to see oneself as separate from thoughts and to just be aware or observe thoughts, rather than react to them. Wells (2005b) gives ten techniques to help promote this skill, such as the free association task. Here, clinicians say a list of neutral words (e.g., dog, chair, gold, blinds, swimming) while patients watch their minds wandering, without attempting to control thoughts at all. As detached mindfulness skills improve, the patients' distressing trigger words are randomly added to the list (e.g., death, failure, ugly, poor) and patients learn to treat them as they would the neutral words.

Another option, used in the treatment protocols of Borkovec et al. (2002), is to practice letting go of worries and training patients' attention on the present moment rather than on the outcomes of past or future events. These therapy components also feature heavily in acceptance and mindfulness-based treatments of GAD, which have demonstrated promising, but preliminary, evidence of therapeutic effects (Craigie et al., 2008; Evans et al., 2008; Hoge et al., 2013; Morgan et al., 2014; Roemer et al., 2008). It is unclear exactly why mindfulness-based interventions are helpful and, like every other treatment component, different theoretical models propose different mechanisms.

"Section 5" of the "Patient treatment manual" in Chapter 6 provides a guide to basic, practical skills for letting go of worries.

Addressing behavioral and avoidance-based symptoms

GAD patients use cognitive and behavioral strategies to control and prevent their worry. Most research has focused on cognitive avoidance and thought-control strategies such as thought suppression and thought replacement. Avoidance behaviors such as avoiding situations that trigger bouts of worry or engaging in safety behaviors (e.g., seeking reassurance, overpreparing, perfectionism) are often reported by patients as a means of preventing and ameliorating worry and its feared consequences. However, the avoidance behaviors associated with GAD have attracted less empirical examination than the cognitive components of GAD and, unlike other anxiety disorders, behaviors are not used to define GAD in the DSM. Nonetheless, behavioral avoidance is elevated in GAD compared to non-clinical populations and greater levels of avoidance at the end of treatment predict poorer outcomes at 6- and 12-month follow-up (Beesdo-Baum et al., 2012). It may therefore be important for patients to learn how to identify and reduce their avoidant behaviors.

Graded exposure Reducing cognitive and behavioral avoidance is a component of all forms of CBT for GAD. The time spent on teaching patients these skills, however, varies across protocols. Some treatment protocols address avoidance in specific sessions (e.g., two to three sessions as Borkovec and Costello (1993), Dugas et al. (2010), and Ost (1987)), whereas others integrate it into the majority of sessions (e.g., as part of behavioral experimentation when testing worries or meta-worries) (Arntz, 2003; Wells, 1997). The rationale for patients learning how to reduce cognitive and behavioral avoidance differs across treatment protocols, as different theoretical accounts argue that avoidance maintains the disorder for different reasons. For example, Wells (1999) argues that chronic reassurance seeking prevents disconfirmation of metacognitive beliefs (e.g., reassurance may stop patients learning that they can control worry or that it is not harmful). Alternatively, the Intolerance of Uncertainty Model of GAD (Dugas et al., 1998) proposes that chronic reassurance seeking prevents patients from learning to tolerate uncertainty.

Patients should be asked about their motivations for engaging in particular forms of avoidance so that clinicians can understand the function of the avoidance for different patients. Returning to our case examples, when Jenny was asked to describe the benefits of not opening her mail, she explained that she felt she could not cope with any problems that might arise from doing so (i.e., signaling negative problem orientation and IU), whereas Tom reported that he phoned his wife frequently to stop his worry about her fidelity overwhelming him (i.e., a negative metacognitive belief).

The rationale for reducing avoidance provided in "Section 6" of the "Patient treatment manual" in Chapter 6 is generic and pertains to testing thoughts and habituating to distressing experiences in a general sense so that clinicians can nominate specific factors relevant to particular patients. A graded exposure and response prevention paradigm is presented to assist patients to cease avoiding worry triggers and using reassurance seeking, thought control, and other safety behaviors.

Unhelpful safety behavior or adaptive coping strategy Clinicians need to examine the function of patients' cognitive and behavioral strategies for managing worry in order to determine if the strategies are unhelpful (i.e., they prevent the disconfirmation of threat appraisals). Some strategies found in the Thought Control Questionnaire (Wells and Davies, 1994), like distraction and social control (e.g., talking to a friend), appear to be more adaptive (Coles and Heimberg, 2005), but it is possible that some patients may use these strategies in unhelpful ways (e.g., seeking excessive reassurance or frantically avoiding distressing thoughts).

Arousal reduction skills (relaxation and breathing control) can also be unhelpful safety behaviors if the patient views them as capable of averting disaster (e.g., believing "If I don't relax and slow my breathing down, I'll lose control of myself"). In this case, the arousal reduction strategies may be preventing the patient from learning that they will not lose control of themselves and that they can cope with distressing feelings.

> Box 5.11 **Safety behaviors: mistakes we have made**
>
> For some patients, we can become a big safety behavior. We can often spot when patients are seeking reassurance from us in face-to-face sessions, but subtle emails and phone calls with questions to "just touch base" have often been our blind spot. The other mistake we often make is setting exposure tasks for our GAD patients. We think we are being helpful by coming up with suggestions, but on lots of occasions, our patients have reported that the exposure was significantly less anxiety-producing because we would never suggest something that was really dangerous, and if anything untoward did happen, we would be responsible for it. Therapist-assisted exposure can also have its traps. For example, following an *in vivo* exposure during a session, a patient once reported that the exercise went very well and then said "and thank goodness you were there to talk to me, it was a great distraction from the worry." This is one of the reasons we use online CBT programs with some of our patients; the computer does not provide reassurance and can foster independence.

See Box 5.11 for common difficulties when addressing safety behaviors.

Imaginal exposure Cognitive avoidance can be addressed by reducing the patient's safety behaviors and avoidance of worry triggers. It is also addressed by imaginal exposure or worry exposure. Imaginal exposure requires patients to confront vivid mental images of their fears and associated thoughts, feelings, and bodily sensations. It is thought that GAD patients avoid these images by worrying and, therefore, fail to adequately process the distressing images. This avoidance inhibits habituation and maintains the patient's anxiety.

It has been argued that imaginal exposure is best employed to address worries that relate to hypothetical future events (Dugas and Ladouceur, 2000). These events are typically highly catastrophic, worst case scenarios that do not easily lend themselves to *in vivo* exposure (e.g., dying in a plane crash, dying alone and destitute). Worry exposure, a form of imaginal exposure, has been successfully used in conjunction with *in vivo* exposure as a stand-alone GAD treatment of approximately 15 weekly sessions (Hoyer et al., 2009).

Worry exposure was first developed by Craske, Barlow, and O'Leary (1992) and is described in "Section 7" of the "Patient treatment manual" in Chapter 6. It involves direct exposure to the image of the patient's worst fear for 25 minutes. The length of time is not empirically derived and acts more as a guide to ensure enough time is given for habituation to the image to occur. The exposure is immediately followed by cognitive restructuring regarding alternative outcomes in order to facilitate changes to the meaning of the feared event (i.e., developing appraisals such as "this event is not likely" or "I could find a way to cope if this happened"). Note that the worry exposure used in the Hoyer et al. (2009) trial did not include any explicit cognitive therapy.

Cognitive exposure is a variant of worry exposure and is a component of IU therapy—three sessions in Dugas et al. (2010); seven sessions in Provencher et al. (2004). Here, patients write a description of their worst case scenario (typically a few minutes long). The idea is to confront the worst or core fear that underlies many of the patient's hypothetical worries. The core fear can be accessed by using the "downward arrow technique" (see Robichaud, 2013, for an illustration). The scenario is recorded on a looped audio tape in the therapy session. The patient then listens to the recording until habituation occurs (generally 20–60 minutes) and repeats this exercise daily (typically for a week or two) until the scenario no longer provokes anxiety and everyday worries related to the scenario subside.

Another variant of worry exposure, similar to that used in the treatment of health anxiety (Furer, Walker, and Stein, 2007), has patients write a story about their worst fear coming true, which they then read and reread for 30 minutes a day. As the exercise is repeated, patients delve deeper into the scenario and their fears. There is some preliminary data to suggest this may be a helpful approach for people who report worrying a lot (Goldman et al., 2007).

One additional clinical application of this technique relates to scheduled "worry time," whereby patients are instructed to "put off" or "save up" their worries throughout the day and channel them (one at a time)

Box 5.12 **Imaginal exposure: mistakes we have made**

By far and away the biggest mistake we have made with worry exposure is not to do it. Imaginal exposure is confronting stuff and, especially in our early years as therapists, we wanted to avoid upsetting and distressing our GAD patients. We felt that we were somehow protecting them when, in actual fact, we were probably perpetuating the worry and reinforcing beliefs that our patients were fragile and vulnerable. To this day, we still walk away from some sessions of worry exposure thinking "that wasn't as bad as I thought it would be" (just like our patients!).

into a 30-minute session when they are free from all other distractions. Subjective levels of anxiety are rated before and after the worry time and, when the 30 minutes are over, patients immediately engage in an absorbing or pleasant activity. The notion is that, over time, patients experience control over the worry and desensitize to the feared scenario.

See Box 5.12 for common difficulties with imaginal exposure.

Therapy tips: Some patients may need training in how to generate vivid, meaningful images that are rich with feelings and sensations (from all five senses). Training can start with practicing imagining pleasant scenarios (e.g., relaxing in a beautiful garden) and move to invoking unpleasant scenes that are unrelated to current worries. Images need to be detailed, specific, and focused on the most frightening aspect of the image (e.g., "having a terminal illness" may be too general, whereas "painfully dying alone in hospital of pancreatic cancer" is better). Other patients can generate highly evocative images, but use safety behaviors to avoid their anxiety (e.g., distracting themselves, seeking reassurance, thinking "it is just a story/ words on a page," avoiding imaginal exposure in specific contexts like at night or when alone). Clinicians may also

Petra: need to monitor any post-exposure neutralizing behaviors (e.g., excessive checking or 'undoing' of the exposure by modifying the image or destroying the paper that it is written on). Adding components of introceptive and *in vivo* exposure may also be useful to enhance the "realness" of the experience (e.g., imagining dying in a bus accident while riding the bus).

Petra: Worry exposure for Petra focused on two particularly distressing images and their associated emotions and core meaning—the "emotional cripple" and the "mad, failed artist." The first one involved the picture of her young self as a hysterical, screaming person who cried, vomited, and passed out while people looked on with horror and disgust at the "freak show." Repeated exposures over several weeks led to reduced anxiety and daily worry as Petra began to see this image as somewhat farcical, ridiculous, and not at all reflecting her current reality and true self. The second image involved her as an old woman, alone and institutionalized, sitting semi-catatonic in a corner, looking at the world go past with black, dead eyes. Petra's anxiety gradually reduced with exposure. The image

---

Box 5.13 Finishing therapy: mistakes we have made

When is enough, enough? We like to think of ourselves as kind and compassionate clinicians, but sometimes we fall into the habit of offering ongoing sessions because a patient is distressed and wants to keep seeing us, even though it is clear that CBT skills are not being practiced and progress is not being made. Continued consultations give both parties the illusion that we are "doing CBT" when we are not. Patients change at different rates, and it is not realistic to expect them to be symptom-free after ten sessions, but we need to remind ourselves that continuing to provide appointments when they result in little benefit is not justified.

persistently evoked sadness but, over time, also led to a feeling of determination that she would not let this happen to her.

Relapse prevention

After cognitive and behavioral skills have been taught and consolidated, *the third stage of treatment* involves planning for the future and preventing symptom relapse. All forms of CBT finish treatment by reviewing the key concepts and skills learned in therapy, and by developing a plan of how to maintain progress and manage the inevitable setbacks and difficulties that will arise in the future. Guidelines on structuring relapse prevention are in "Section 8" of the "Patient treatment manual" in Chapter 6.

See Box 5.13 for common difficulties when finishing therapy.

Summary

CBT for GAD begins with assessment and formulation. Treatment involves three broad stages—psychoeducation and treatment rationale, skill development and consolidation, and relapse prevention. The order of and emphasis placed on different skills may vary across patients, but it is likely that most patients will find the majority of skills helpful to some extent.

Chapter 6

Patient treatment manual

Hello and welcome! Congratulations on having the courage to tackle your anxiety and take control of your worry. This program will explain what generalized anxiety disorder (GAD) is and how you can manage it.

The program is based on cognitive behavior therapy (CBT) which is an effective treatment for anxiety. Learning to manage worry is a skill and, like any skill, it needs to be practiced regularly to be effective.

Here is what people with GAD have said about this program:

* Sharise (36)—"It was such a relief to get some practical strategies to help me get my worry under control."

* Chen (23)—"Doing this program, I realized I wasn't the only one with anxiety, and there was something I could do about it ... not just take a pill, but do something myself."

* Kala (59)—"I feel good about myself again! I still have a long way to go, but I know I'll get better if I just keep working on it."

Here is an overview of the program:

Section 1 Understanding generalized anxiety disorder
Section 2 Understanding what keeps your worry going
Section 3 Managing physical symptoms
Section 4 Managing thinking symptoms
Section 5 Advanced skills for managing worry thoughts
Section 6 Dealing with behaviors that affect worry
Section 7 Advanced skills for facing fears
Section 8 Putting it all together and staying well in the longer term

This program is very detailed. There is a list of frequently asked questions at the end of this manual to help you navigate through the program (see Table 6.17). You may prefer to work through this course on your own or with your clinician.

The early sections will take you about a week or two to work through, but allow several weeks to fully work through each of the skills in

Sections 4–7. However, it is important to complete the program at your own pace. Blank copies of every form used are in the back of this manual. Please reproduce them as needed.

Throughout this program, you will meet someone who has GAD. Her name is Liz. As you read about her experiences, you will learn how to manage your own anxiety. You may not relate to everything Liz experiences, because everyone is unique, but we hope you will enjoy this program and learn some useful skills for managing your worry. Let us meet Liz …

> Hi, nice to meet you! I've been a big worrier for as long as I can remember. I used to think it was the way everyone thought but about a year ago, I lost my job, and the worry got really bad. When I found a new job, I expected the worry to go away … it didn't. So I decided I needed to do something about it.

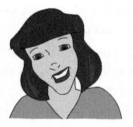

Section 1: UNDERSTANDING GENERALIZED ANXIETY DISORDER

What is generalized anxiety disorder?

Generalized anxiety disorder (GAD) is a type of anxiety disorder which involves persistent worry and feelings of anxiety about a variety of everyday concerns such as family, work, health, finances, safety, and relationships.

> I think I understand … but what exactly do you mean by "worry"?

Worry is a stream of thoughts or ideas in your head about future events which are negative or uncertain, and lead to feelings of apprehension or anxiety. One way to think about worry is as a type of "self-talk" where you are having a conversation in your head about what might happen in the future and how you would deal with that. Worries often come in the form of "what if ..."

> Oh like ... What if I get fired? What if the kids get really sick? What if I am not a good enough wife? What if my friends stop liking me?

Is GAD rare?

No, GAD is one of the more common anxiety disorders. About 2 in 100 people experience it in any given year. So, if you think you are experiencing GAD, be assured, you are not alone!

But everyone worries—how is GAD different?

Yes, everyone worries—particularly during stressful life events. However, after the stress resolves, the worry and anxiety generally subsides. The worry in GAD is very different. It is:

+ Excessive—out of proportion to the circumstances you are experiencing. You may feel like you make a "mountain out of a mole hill" or are always "thinking the worst" when the worst rarely occurs.

+ Difficult to control— hard to "turn off" the worry, even when there does not seem to be anything to be anxious about.

+ Pervasive and persistent—the worry always seems to be around. It is intrusive and spreads to lots of areas in your life. For a diagnosis, the worry and anxiety need to be there more days than not for at least 6 months, but many people with GAD feel they have been a worrier for many years ... if not their whole life.

> I know how that feels ... so many people have told me to "just stop worrying" ... as if it were that easy! It can be really frustrating when people don't understand how difficult it is.

The worry in GAD is also:

- Associated with symptoms such as muscle tension; fatigue; difficulty concentrating and sleeping; feeling irritable, restless, keyed up, and on edge.

- Distressing and disabling—it is difficult to do things you want to do. You may struggle with procrastination or perfectionism, or avoid doing things because you feel unsure or overwhelmed.

Liz, how does GAD affect your life?

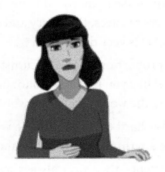

Form 6.1 What areas of your life does GAD interfere with?

Check the boxes that apply to you:

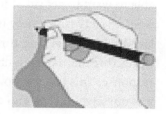

☐ It interferes with my personal life

☐ It interferes with my job/education/
career

☐ It affects how I get on with others

☐ It affects how I feel about myself

☐ It stops me doing things I want to do

☐ It affects my health

Note down other areas here:

How do I get rid of the worry and anxiety?

When worry is so distressing and debilitating, it is entirely understandable to want to get rid of it altogether. However, let us think a bit about what anxiety is. Anxiety is a normal emotional reaction. When we are faced with something threatening, or when we anticipate that something threatening may happen, our body reacts with the fight/flight response. This is our automatic fear response and it prepares us to protect ourselves (i.e., to run away or fight).

The fight/flight response leads to a host of important physical changes. Put yourself in this situation— you are sitting in a garden when you hear some rustling behind you and out of the corner of your eye you see something small and black scuttling closer to you. Your brain becomes aware of danger. Automatically, hormones are released and the involuntary nervous system sends signals to various parts of the body to produce a number of important changes. These changes allow you to rapidly move away from the spider:

- Your heart rate speeds up and blood pressure rises (you feel tense, your heart beats faster).
- You breathe quicker. Your nostrils and the air passages in your lungs open wider to allow air in more quickly (you may feel dizzy, light-headed, or unwell).
- Your mind becomes alert and focussed on the source of the threat.
- You may sweat more to help cool your body.
- Blood is diverted to your muscles, which tense, ready for action (your hands may feel cold and clammy, or you may feel shaky or restless).
- Your digestion slows down (you may feel sick or have "butterflies" in your stomach).
- Saliva production decreases, causing a dry mouth.
- Blood clotting ability increases, preparing for possible injury.
- The liver releases sugar to provide quick energy.

• Sphincter muscles contract to close the openings of the bowel and bladder.

Do these feelings sound familiar? You may have similar feelings when you worry. The fight/flight response is useful in the short term, especially if the danger can be dealt with by physical exertion.

Anxiety can also help you perform well. It is motivating and can enhance your efficiency. If you are completely relaxed when you attend a job interview, play sport, or go on a date, you may not be able to do your best. To do anything really well, you need to be alert, focussed, and motivated. Anxiety, in moderation, can be helpful.

> So anxiety is a matter of degree—I've got to get the balance right. It's good to feel alert and a bit tense, like when I'm chairing a meeting at work, but I've got to learn to master my anxiety when it is excessive.
> I feel irritable and on edge a lot. It's like my fight/flight response is triggered off all the time . . . even when nothing bad is happening.

The fight/flight response is triggered whenever you *perceive or anticipate* danger—whether it is truly there or not. Dangers do not have to be physical threats, like poisonous spiders; they can be things like being rejected or making mistakes at work. The problem is that many of the things people with GAD worry about do not come to pass, so the fight/flight response is a little like a false alarm going off.

Although the fight/flight response is not dangerous, it can feel uncomfortable and unpleasant. Sometimes these feelings can trigger more worry, especially if they seem to come out of the blue.

> Sometimes I worry about why I feel so churned up inside . . . I think, I've got cancer or I'm going to faint or be sick . . . maybe the churning feeling is just my fight/flight response?

What causes GAD?

We do not know what definitively causes GAD, but research has identified some factors that seem to make people more vulnerable to developing problems with excessive worry and anxiety. For most people with GAD, it will be a combination of factors.

Although there does not appear to be a specific gene for GAD, people may inherit a general vulnerability to anxiety and mood disorders—that is, these difficulties tend to run in families.

People who are born with an anxious and sensitive type of temperament may also be predisposed to developing an anxiety disorder.

We also think that experiencing difficult life events may combine with genetic vulnerabilities to increase a person's chance of developing problems with anxiety. Events that are particularly stressful, painful, traumatic, or uncontrollable may affect the way a person views themselves, their relationships, and the world. For example, coming to believe that bad things will happen to you, the world is a dangerous place, and that other people are unpredictable. Our world view is often influenced by other people, like our parents, siblings, and friends. You may have been taught from a young age to be wary or fearful of particular things, or you may have observed your family members being overly anxious.

> That sounds like me ... I have always been a bit of a worrier ... so has my dad and sister

What can I do about this worry and anxiety?

There are several treatments for GAD. The main effective ones are medications (a specific group called selective serotonin re-uptake inhibitors (SSRIs) or antidepressants) and a type of psychotherapy called cognitive behavioral therapy (CBT). The aim of CBT is to help you identify and shift unhelpful thoughts and behaviors that keep excessive worry going. This manual is based on CBT.

If your doctor has prescribed you medication, it is important that you continue to take the medication for several months, and only stop taking it in consultation with your doctor.

> But I heard that medication is addictive and that it can change your personality or make you feel really out of it!

No, that is not the case. This type of medication is safe. Side-effects, such as an upset stomach, sleep problems, and restlessness, usually settle over time, and can be minimized by starting on a low dose and then gradually increasing. If you experience side-effects on one medicine, your doctor may suggest another, as they differ in how they affect individuals. These medications are not addictive. That said, when you are ready to stop the medication, people benefit from gradually reducing the dose.

A special note on sedatives, tranquilizers, and sleeping pills

Sometimes people use sedative medications. These medications are useful for short periods (e.g., for 1–2 weeks), but are not recommended for long-term use. The benzodiazepines, particularly Xanax, are addictive drugs. They have been associated with clouded thinking, risk of falls, and traffic accidents. If you are taking these medications, see your doctor to discuss slowly decreasing the dose and ceasing them. These medications interfere with a program like this one because they prevent you from mastering your anxiety. The same is true of alcohol. Over time, these substances actually make anxiety worse.

Section 2: UNDERSTANDING WHAT KEEPS YOUR WORRY GOING

There are three types of symptoms in GAD:

- Thoughts (e.g., your ideas, beliefs, worries … all the "self-talk" that runs through your mind) and thinking processes (like attention and memory)
- Physical symptoms
- Behaviors (i.e., the things you do to manage the worry and anxiety)

These symptoms can be triggered by specific situations, or they can seem to just "come out of the blue." The symptoms interact with each other to keep the problem going. Let us look at an example from Liz's experience (see Figure 6.1).

> I often get worried at work. When I look at my diary (trigger situation) I often start to worry "How will I get through all this? Sooner or later, my boss will find out I can't do this job … that I'm a fraud" (thoughts). I tense up and start to get a headache (physical symptoms). Then I think "I'm making myself sick with all this worry" (thoughts). So, I subtly check with my assistant that we are on top of everything and go over the plans for the day and how he needs to remind me to do everything to make sure we keep the boss happy (behaviors). All this planning and preparing makes me restless and edgy, and my headache gets worse (physical symptoms), so I fiddle around on the internet for a while before getting started with my work (behaviors), until I start to worry I am running out of time to finish my reports (thoughts).

In Figure 6.1, notice how the symptoms interact to keep the problem going. The worries lead to the physical symptoms and checking behaviors, and then the headaches and procrastination lead to more worry. Thus the cycle continues around and around.

Trigger situation

Looking at my calendar at work

Thoughts

How will I get through all this? My boss will find out I can't do this job and think I'm a fraud!

I'm making myself sick with all this worry!

I'm running out of time to finish my reports!

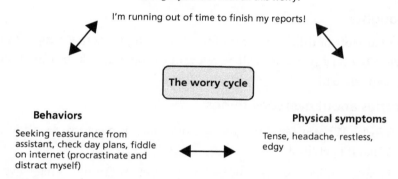

Figure 6.1 Liz's worry cycle.

Triggering situations

Liz started to worry in a variety situations. Some triggers were specific situations ...

> When I watch the news, I worry about being attacked or our house being burgled. Or if I drive past the hospital, I start to worry about getting sick or dying one day. I also worry at work, or when I have to make decisions or hand in my reports.

Other triggers for Liz's worry were internal experiences ...

> I worry if my heart skips a beat or if I feel faint and dizzy ... I know it is silly, but I start to worry that I have a brain tumor. Or sometimes, out of the blue, I get scary images in my head of my children being hurt, or my partner being in a car accident. At other times, my worry is triggered by a funny feeling of things just not being right ... like a sense of dread comes over me.

Think about what triggers your bouts of worry and note them down here. It may be specific situations or when you are around specific people, or it may be certain feelings, images, or bodily sensations.

_____

_____

_____

_____

Thoughts

There are lots of different types of thinking symptoms that people can have. Not every symptom will be relevant to you, but tick the ones that you can relate to.

Worries about everyday things

☐ Work—What if I cannot get my work done or meet my deadlines? What if I get fired?

☐ Family—What if something bad happens to my family? What if everyone cannot get along better?

☐ Health—What if I have cancer/ heart disease/ dementia/ a terrible infection? This is not normal; there must be something very wrong with me.

☐ Mental health—I am always going to be anxious; I will never be "normal." What if I am psychotic/ mad/ insane? I cannot concentrate and it is affecting my whole life.

☐ Future—What will happen in the future? What if I am unhappy? What if my children do not like me? What if I have made the wrong decisions and have lots of regrets? What if I never get better?

☐ Everyday activities—Worries about being on time, being polite, losing things, etc.

☐ Social situations—What if people do not like me or want to be around me? Everyone thinks I am crazy/ stupid/ weak/ pathetic/ a loser. What if no one can understand what I am going through?

☐ Catastrophes—What if the house burns down? My child is kidnapped? I end up destitute? My partner dies in a car accident?

☐ Finances—I will not have enough money to pay my bills. What if I have not made the right financial decisions? I cannot cope with all my debt.

☐ Safety—What if I get attacked? What if my house gets broken into?

☐ World affairs—Worry about wars, crimes, poverty, politics, the environment, etc.

☐ Failure— I will never be able to do this right. I am hopeless/ useless/ not good enough.

☐ Perfectionism—Things will be awful if they are not 100%. If things are not perfect, it is not good enough. There is no point doing things if they will not be perfect.

☐ Coping—I can never cope. Others are always better at dealing with problems. I cannot handle it when bad things happen.

☐ Problem solving— I am no good at solving problems; things never work out for me. Other people are much better at making decisions; I just get overwhelmed and do not know what to do.

☐ Uncertainties— If I do not know what is going to happen, I cannot cope. It is best to be 100% sure before you do anything. Anything could happen; I need to be prepared.

Worries about worries

Often people with GAD worry about their worry—which naturally makes worry more distressing and perpetuates the worry cycle. Have you ever thought that:

☐ I could get into a state of worrying and never be able to stop.

☐ If I worry too much, I could lose control.

☐ If I do not control my worry, then it will control me.

☐ If I worry it means I am a weak person.

☐ My worry is harmful to others.

☐ My worry is uncontrollable—it is taking over me and I cannot stop it.

☐ My worry is dangerous.

☐ Worrying is harmful to me.

☐ Worrying makes me sick.

☐ My worry will never end.

☐ Worry could make me go crazy.

☐ My worry is ruining my relationships.

> Lots of these sound familiar! I tend to make things into a catastrophe. What a mountain of worry thoughts. I never realized how many worries I had. My fight/flight response must be working overtime ... no wonder I get headaches!

Believing worry is good

You may also have beliefs about how your worry could be helpful or advantageous. Tick the thoughts you have had:

☐ Worrying helps me to cope.

☐ Worry stops everything falling apart.

☐ Worry helps me get things done.

☐ My worries are realistic and very likely to happen.

☐ Worrying keeps me safe.

☐ Without my worry, I would not know what to do.

☐ Worry helps me cope when I do not know what will happen.

☐ Worrying stops bad things from happening.

☐ Worrying motivates me to do things.

☐ Worry helps me to check on my health.

☐ Worry stops me making mistakes/ getting into trouble.

☐ Worrying helps me to be prepared for all possibilities.

☐ Worrying helps me to solve problems.

☐ Worrying shows I care.

☐ Worry prevents me from offending people.

☐ Worry prepares me for the worst.

Thinking processes

It is not just what you think but *how* you think that can keep anxiety going. Anxious people tend to pay attention to and remember threatening information. That is, there may be a bias towards or filter on what you focus on and the experiences you recall. It is as though you are wearing 'doom and gloom glasses' and seeing all the dangerous or bad things, and dismissing positive or reassuring experiences. Over time these biases reinforce and strengthen your fears, so you need to learn to recognize when you are wearing the doom and gloom glasses.

Physical symptoms

Consider the physical symptoms you experience when you worry. Tick the ones that apply to you:

☐ Heart palpitations, pounding heart

☐ Blushing

☐ Sweating, clammy hands

☐ Feeling short of breath, feeling like you cannot get enough air

☐ Trembling or shaking

☐ Feeling dizzy, light-headed, faint, or unsteady

☐ Muscle tension

☐ Headaches

☐ Feeling on edge or keyed up

> When I get these physical symptoms, I worry more. For example, I think "people will think I am weird if they see me flustered" or "I feel so unwell, something must be seriously wrong with me." Sometimes I get angry with myself; I tell myself it is selfish and stupid to get so worked up.

The thinking and feeling symptoms of GAD are unpleasant, so it is no surprise that people with GAD do many things to avoid or prevent the worry.

Behaviors

Avoidance is very common in GAD. Although it can reduce your anxiety in the short term, it actually keeps the worry cycle going. It does this by preventing you from finding out:

1. If the thing you are worried about actually happens, and

2. How you cope when unexpected or unpleasant things happen.

> Oh, so when I avoid opening the mail or answering the phone, I don't get the chance to find out that it is not bad news, and if it were, I could find a way to cope? That makes sense.

Avoidance can lead to even more problems. Liz, what happens when you avoid answering phone calls and opening the mail?

> Well, my friends get annoyed that they can never reach me. Also, sometimes I don't pay bills or file away bank letters correctly … then I get all flustered and worried.

So avoidance actually makes the problem worse and undermines your ability to cope. Let us have a look at your avoidance behaviors. Often people avoid the things that trigger their worry—like the things you wrote down in the "Triggering situations" section.

> I avoid exercise because it makes my heart race and my head spin. I also avoid watching TV shows about hospitals or reading news articles about crimes. At work, I procrastinate if I am worried about handing in a report or having a meeting with my boss. It just makes everything worse, but it seems easier at the time. Sometimes I avoid socializing or talking to people at work—I worry I might say something stupid or embarrassing.

Make a list of the things you avoid:

_____

_____

_____

_____

Sometimes we cannot completely avoid things, so people often develop a raft of subtle avoidance behaviors. These are called "safety behaviors" because people believe that the behavior will help them cope or prevent their fears from coming true.

I know what you mean. I worry that my boss will think my work is not good enough. So when I can't get out of a meeting with her, I spend hours preparing for it, and I check and double check my reports. During the meeting, I spend a lot of time trying to figure out if she is happy with my work. I'm always trying to please other people and get their approval.

The problem is that safety behaviors only provide an illusion of control. You can become dependent on them and fail to discover that you can cope on your own. Common safety behaviors include (tick the ones you use):

☐ Overplanning—always having a "plan B" (and plan C, D, E, F …)

☐ Excessive list making

☐ Seeking constant reassurance from others (including family, friends, doctors, and other information sources like the internet) that your fears are not true

☐ Seeking reassurance from yourself (e.g., by replaying events over and over in your mind, checking your body excessively, checking and rechecking that you have done things correctly)

☐ Excessively controlling situations or people

☐ Deferring decisions to others

☐ Seeking approval from others

☐ Procrastinating

☐ Closely monitoring what you think, say, and do

☐ Cutting activities short

☐ Checking up on other people a lot (e.g., calling and emailing to make sure they are OK)

☐ Acting very carefully and cautiously

☐ Being unable to say no or give your opinion

☐ Being a perfectionist

☐ Having companions to avoid doing things alone

☐ Taking on other people's responsibilities (or abdicating your responsibilities to others)

☐ Talking too much to avoid awkward silences

☐ Pretending not to notice people you know

☐ Sitting at the back of the room so people do not notice you

☐ Superstitious behaviors (touching wood, saying special words, "undoing" things in your mind)

There is one last form of avoidance that I would like to mention and that has to do with controlling thoughts. Remember those "worry about worry" thoughts? We are talking about beliefs such as "worry is dangerous and could make me go mad." People with GAD sometimes use particular safety behaviors to control or limit their worry in order to prevent their fears (like the fear of going mad from worry) from coming true.

These unhelpful thought-control strategies may include (tick the ones relevant to you):

☐ Thought suppression (i.e., pushing worries away or telling yourself to stop worrying)

☐ Debating with the worry (e.g., telling yourself "that couldn't happen because …")

☐ Unhelpful distraction (i.e., occupying your mind with activities because you want to prevent a disaster, like going mad)

☐ Being self-critical or punishing yourself (e.g., telling yourself you are stupid and foolish for worrying)

☐ Replacing worries with overly positive thoughts (e.g., "I'll not fail my test—I'll get 100%")

☐ Replacing big worries with more minor ones (e.g., "I won't think about our bills, I'll just worry about cooking the chicken for tonight")

What's so wrong with these strategies … don't I want to stop worrying?

Great question! Using these strategies can be unhelpful when they prevent you finding out if your fears are true (e.g., can worry really send me mad?) or if you can cope without them (do I need to frantically distract myself, or can I learn to get on with my day despite the worry popping back into my mind from time to time?).

These strategies can also have nasty rebound effects. For example, overly positive thoughts can feel like you are just fooling yourself. Thought suppression is also problematic because the more you try not to think something, the more likely you are to think about it. In order not to think about something, *we actually have to think about not thinking about it*. So, in fact, we are ultra-vigilant to the thought and think it more and more!

You can do an amusing experiment to experience this rebound effect. For the next minute, do not think about pink elephants … whatever you do, do not think about pink elephants. What happens?

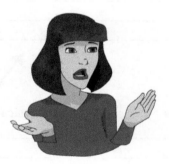

I'm thinking about pink elephants … I wasn't thinking about them before, but now I am trying not to think about them, they pop back into my mind!

There are ways to manage worrying thoughts so that they do not get worse and worse. However, before we go further, let us put all these elements together to create your own worry cycle.

Form 6.2 Your worry cycle

Look back over this section and write in your trigger situations, worry thoughts, physical symptoms, and behaviors.

Trigger situations

_____

_____

_____

_____

_____

⇩

Thoughts

_____

_____

_____

_____

_____

_____

Behaviors   **Physical symptoms**

_____   _____

_____   _____

_____   _____

_____   _____

> There seems so much I need to change to take control of my worry … It's overwhelming! I don't think I can do it. I've relied on avoidance and safety behaviors for so long … I don't think I could cope without them. It's hopeless!

Slow down Liz. When you feel overwhelmed, it is helpful to break tasks down into more manageable pieces. You do not need to change everything all at once. Little by little, you will learn new ways to respond to worrying situations. Changes in one area (e.g., physical symptoms) often reduce symptoms in other areas (e.g., thought symptoms). Do not give up—you *can* make a meaningful difference to your life!

How does cognitive behavior therapy (CBT) break the cycle apart?

CBT breaks down the worry cycle by addressing the three types of symptoms of GAD. One of the key ideas in this program is learning to experiment or test out your worrying thoughts and behaviors. We do not expect you to believe us when we say that doing certain things is not harmful. We want you to find things out for yourself! At the same time, we do not want you to assume that your worries are 100% true. Again, we want you to test this out for yourself.

The best way to do this is to experiment. The problem with worrying and avoiding things is that doing so stops you from testing if your fears are accurate. Worrying and avoiding things also stops you from improving your ability to cope with difficult situations and feelings. During this program, we really encourage you to be curious and to give the skills and strategies a decent trial.

Discovery exercises

For the next week or so, pay attention to how your worry operates—be curious and note what the worry does and how it keeps going. The best way to do this is to monitor your worries using a log.

Table 6.1 is a sample from Liz's monitoring. (A blank log for you can be found towards the back of this manual; see Form 6.3.) Part of monitoring worry is learning to assess how strong your feelings are in

Table 6.1 Liz's worry log

Date and situation	Feelings and physical symptoms What did I feel and what happened in my body?	Thoughts What went through my mind?	Behaviors What did I do?
Thursday 6 pm, waiting for John	Anxious (90/100) Irritated (70/100) Heart racing, tense, shaky (80/100)	Where is John? Why is he not home? What if he has had an accident? How would I cope?	Call John's work, call his mobile phone, look on news for any accident reports.
Saturday 3.30 pm; preparing for dinner guests	Anxious (85/100) Hopeless (50/100) Sore neck, on edge, headache, short of breath (60/100)	What if they do not like the food? The house is such a mess! I never know what to say—everyone will think I am a terrible host.	Seek reassurance from John, clean the house for hours, prepare food in advance, think up conversations I can make.

anxiety-producing situations. This is generally done by subjectively rating your feelings from 0 to 100, where 0 is no feeling and 100 is the maximum feeling possible.

> I really found this exercise helpful—I thought I knew everything about my worry, but doing this detective work was a real eye-opener. I started to see how the worry crept into lots of areas of my life, and how I was so quick to jump to the worst case scenario. I also become a lot more aware of my safety behaviors which actually made it easier for me to drop them off.

Section 3: MANAGING PHYSICAL SYMPTOMS

This section looks at skills you can learn to help manage the physical symptoms of GAD.

Controlled breathing

Recall that when we become worried or anxious our breathing rate can speed up. This is part of the fight/flight response. Hyperventilation occurs when we breathe too quickly or deeply than our body needs. It can lead to many uncomfortable symptoms like dizziness, confusion, numbness, nausea, tingling, breathlessness, and tension. If you want to demonstrate this to yourself, deliberately breathe deeply and quickly for a handful of breaths or until you start to notice the sensations build up.

> That wasn't a fun exercise . . . it only took three deep, fast breaths before I felt dizzy and sick!

You may be overbreathing when you become anxious, or you may be overbreathing most of the time without being aware of it. Do a quick test now—use a watch with a second hand (or timer) and count the number of breaths you take over one minute (where one breath is in and out).

Write it here: _____ breaths per minute

> Mine was 16.

A normal resting breathing rate is 10–12 breaths per minute.

> Maybe I am breathing a bit too quickly, then.

Does it matter where you breathe from?

Many people who overbreathe tend to breathe with their chest muscles rather than their diaphragm, and these muscles can become tight and sore. When you breathe, breathe from your tummy and through the nose, consciously attempting to breathe in a smooth and gentle way.

I think I do hyperventilate a bit … is it dangerous?

Not at all, but it can make you more likely to feel apprehensive, slightly dizzy, and unable to think clearly. One way of managing the physical symptoms of your anxiety is to regularly use controlled breathing. The aim is to use it at times during the day when you notice you are starting to feel distressed, anxious, or worried. However remember, slow, controlled breathing is not deep breathing. Breathing too deeply is a form of hyperventilation.

If you would like to try some controlled breathing, follow this exercise:

Step 1. Sit comfortably in a chair. Use a watch with a second hand to time yourself. Breathe in and out gently through your nose. Rest your hands on your tummy to check that you are using your stomach muscles (and therefore, your diaphragm) to drive your breathing, rather than your upper chest.

Step 2. Now, do the following exercise:
Breathe in for 3 seconds, pause, and breathe out for 3 seconds.
As you breathe out, relax your body (and say the word "relax" to yourself). Do this for 3 minutes and notice the difference in your tension or anxiety. Try counting your breathing rate for 1 minute, before and after the exercise. Does your breathing rate drop afterwards?
Write it here: _____breaths per minute

The controlled breathing exercise can be done at different times throughout the day. At first, you may need to find a quiet, relaxing place. With practice, it becomes easier and you can use it whenever you need to.

Some people find that they feel a little anxious or uncomfortable when they first start controlled breathing. This may be due to breathing a little fast or becoming sensitive to breathing patterns when you think about them. It is normal for this skill to feel odd at first. As you practice the slow breathing technique, it will feel more natural.

Optional extra!

There are many varieties of controlled breathing techniques. If the "3 in, 3 out" does not feel good to you, try something else. Some people like to breathe in for 4 seconds, hold for 2 seconds, and then breathe out for 6 seconds; or breathe in for 3, hold for 2, and 5 out ... just experiment and see what works best for you!

Relaxation training

Our muscles tense up when we are anxious or stressed—again, another part of the fight/flight response. Unfortunately, long periods of muscle tension can cause muscle pain, headaches, and fatigue. Ongoing muscle tension may also contribute to the feelings of constant apprehension, irritability, and jumpiness.

One way to manage this tension is by learning how to recognize and reduce excess tension. We will introduce you to one technique called Progressive Muscle Relaxation (PMR).

The PMR technique involves tensing and relaxing the major muscle groups in your body in a systematic manner. You can do this by following the set of exercises at the end of this manual. Over time, you will learn the sequence and will not need to keep referring to the scripted procedure. Some people prefer to be guided through the exercises by listening to a recording (e.g., you can purchase a CD or download an audio file from the internet).

Ideally, relaxation training should be practiced daily for two months or longer. Some people feel distressed and anxious during relaxation exercises. You may feel that you are "wasting time" or just not used to feeling relaxed. Remind yourself that relaxation training is a valuable use of time because it will assist you in your recovery. If you are not used to feeling relaxed, this is all the more reason to keep practicing—in time, you will start to find relaxation training an enjoyable and beneficial exercise.

It often helps to keep a log of your experiences so you can see how you progress. There is a log to use at the end of this manual (see Form 6.4).

You can try PMR in the evening, to improve your sleep, or use it to help you relax if you wake up worrying throughout the night.

Exercise

Exercise can help manage low mood and worry. It can help you shift your attention away from worries and use up "nervous energy." Exercise also releases endorphins which can boost your mood.

We recommend that you aim for 30 minutes of moderate exercise most days. On a couple of days, try some more vigorous exercise (the kind that makes you huff and puff) with some strengthening exercises (e.g., lifting weights or doing sit-ups).

Tips for exercise

- Pick an exercise goal—stick to it! If your goal is walking for 15 minutes three times a week, that is great. If your goal is to swim 40 laps of the pool, that is great, too. The important thing is to choose a goal and stick to it!

- Be accountable! Is there someone who can exercise with you, or help you stay on track?

- On some days, accumulate your 30 minutes a day by combining shorter sessions—like a 10-minute walk with the dog, mowing the lawn, or cycling with the kids to the park.

- Pick a task that you can succeed at and that you enjoy. If you are not confident to run for 30 minutes, go for a 10-minute walk instead.

- Exercise regularly and consistently. Make time in your week to exercise, rather than exercise if the opportunity arises.

- Pick a number of different tasks that can suit a variety of times and conditions. Do not miss your exercise target just because it is raining, or too hot, or a venue is booked out.

- See your doctor if you have any health complaints. Doctors and physiotherapists can often recommend exercise you can do even if you have a medical condition.

- If you stop— just start again! Do not beat yourself up about stopping. Think about what you have done and can do, and turn this into what you will do—and start again!

- Build in some rewards to congratulate yourself for your hard work and to motivate you.

> So many things to do ... I just don't have the time to do all this breathing and relaxing and exercising! I'll never get better!
>
> Hang on; it helps to break things down. I'll just start by doing a little bit as part of my normal routine. I catch the train to work ... I'll do the relaxation and breathing then. I might have time to do them before I go to bed as well.
>
> But I hate exercise ... how can I make that easier? What if I didn't drive to mum's on Tuesdays ... I could walk instead ... that would be about 20 minutes.

Great work Liz! Most people find it very hard to make time for themselves and to put these new skills into place.

> But if I don't do anything, nothing will change, and I can't keep living with all this worry and anxiety!

That is true. Give these skills a decent try for the next few weeks. When you notice that you are feeling anxious, try the controlled breathing and relaxation. However, remember to be patient with yourself. You may have been anxious for many years, and it will take time and lots of persistent effort to overcome your worry habits.

Do not be too discouraged when you have setbacks along the way. They are normal; everyone has them. The road to recovery is a bumpy one (see Figure 6.2). Remember that setbacks are temporary; they will not last. So keep using the skills in this manual, and do not give up!

For the next week, we would like you to keep going with the discovery exercises from Section 1. We would also like you to try the controlled breathing, relaxation, and exercise skills. Good luck and we will see you again soon!

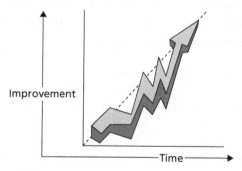

Figure 6.2 Setbacks are normal.

Section 4: MANAGING THINKING SYMPTOMS

This section addresses worrying thoughts associated with everyday situations, coping with problems, and dealing with uncertain events. It is a big section and may take several weeks to work through.

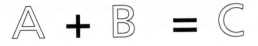

An event   Belief/thought   Consequence:
emotion and behavior

Figure 6.3 The ABC Model.

Worrying thoughts are an important part of the worry cycle. There is a relationship between what we think and how we feel. We call this relationship the "ABC Model" (see Figure 6.3). The "A" stands for an event or situation, "B" is a thought or belief, and "C" is a consequence (the emotion).

We often assume that situations (A) determine how we feel (C). However, according to the ABC Model, it is the way we think about the situation (B) that influences how we feel and what we do (C).

Thoughts are important because they affect the way we feel

Let us consider an example. You are meeting a friend for coffee at 3.00 pm. It is now 3.20 pm. You are waiting at the café and your friend has not arrived. Three people in the same situation have entirely different thoughts and feelings (see Table 6.2).

> That sounds familiar—I'd be like Person 1 or 2. I'd think the worst and get all worked up!

Table 6.2 Thoughts influence how you feel and what you do (example 1)

	Thoughts	**Feelings and behaviors**
Person 1	"Oh no, my friend must have been in an accident!"	Anxious and worried Try to phone friend
Person 2	"My friend isn't coming because they don't like me anymore. I've been stood up."	Angry, hurt, and depressed Go home
Person 3	"My friend has probably been held up at work and will probably be here soon."	Neutral, mild irritation Order a coffee, start reading a magazine

Table 6.3 Thoughts influence how you feel and what you do (example 2)

	Thoughts	**Feelings and behaviors**
Person 1	"It must be a burglar!"	Anxious and frightened Wake up partner
Person 2	"It was just the cat next door jumping down from the fence."	Neutral, mild irritation Go back to sleep
Person 3	"My neighbor is deliberately trying to make noise so I don't sleep!"	Annoyed Dwell on things you would like to say to your neighbor

Let us consider another example. You are lying in bed one night and hear a loud thump outside. Again, different people may have different thoughts and feelings (see Table 6.3).

These simple examples illustrate that the way we interpret a situation has a big impact upon the way we feel. Often, we assume that it is the situation itself that causes us to feel a certain way. In fact, it is the *way we think about the situation that really affects the way we feel about it.* This can influence what we do, and our actions can then impact on our thoughts or beliefs. Sometimes, our thoughts can become a self-fulfilling prophecy! Here are some examples (see Table 6.4).

Our thoughts and the way we interpret particular situations are shaped through our present and past experiences and our knowledge, values, culture, and upbringing. Because of this, and because they tend to occur automatically, they are very *believable.* The problem with this is

Table 6.4 Thoughts can become self-fulfilling

Thought	**Feeling and action**	**Self-fulfillment**
I am a failure	Depressed—stay in bed most of the day, drink too much wine, be self-critical	By achieving very little during the day, I end up believing I am more of a failure
People will think I am stupid and boring	Nervous—do not say much around people, avoid eye contact	People tend not to talk to me for very long, so I end up believing I really am stupid and boring
This treatment will not work	Hopeless—avoid doing therapy tasks, cancel appointments with my doctor, forget to take medication	Nothing in my life changes and I doubt more than ever that anything will help me feel better

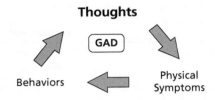

Figure 6.4 Biased thinking can maintain anxiety.

that we often assume that our thoughts are accurate, and never question whether they are true, helpful, or valid.

In GAD, our thoughts can become biased and help to maintain the anxiety (see Figure 6.4). You may often think about bad things happening, when other people do not seem to be worried.

The good thing about thoughts is that they can be changed and shifted. They are not facts; they can be altered over time. We can step back from our thoughts to examine their accuracy and helpfulness. If you can think differently about worrying situations, then you are more likely to feel less distressed.

Unhelpful thinking patterns

It is important to recognize GAD thinking symptoms. By now, you will have identified a variety of worrying thoughts through your monitoring exercises. You may also want to take a look at the worry thoughts you selected in Section 2 of this manual. Do you notice any patterns or themes in the sorts of things you worry about?

Often, people engage in unhelpful thinking patterns or common thinking errors. We can call them errors because they are biased or prejudiced ways of interpreting situations that often do not take into account all the facts. Let us take a look at the common errors (tick the ones you experience):

☐ **Jumping to conclusions:** Drawing a conclusion without any evidence to support the conclusion. For example, "I have a bit of a sore throat … it must be cancer."

☐ **Mind reading:** You automatically assume that you know that someone is thinking negatively about you without checking this out with them. For example, a colleague walks past your office and does not say hello. You assume, "They think I'm boring and don't want to talk to me."

☐ **Selective thinking (mental filter/mental bias):** This is when you focus on a detail taken out of context and ignore other more important aspects of the situation. For example, after not receiving a phone call from a friend you conclude, "They don't really care about me."

☐ **Catastrophizing:** This refers to the tendency to turn situations into life or death. Your imagination creates images of disasters that have not happened and are unlikely to happen. For example, you hand in a report and realize it had a spelling mistake. You then worry that your boss will think you are incompetent. You then start to think you will be fired and that your boss will give you a bad reference so that you will never be able to get another job again … and so on!

☐ **Personalizing ("it's all my fault"):** This refers to the tendency to relate situations to yourself when there is no basis for making such a connection. You see yourself as the cause of some negative event for which, in fact, you were not primarily responsible. For example, your boss storms into his office and slams the door and you think, "What have I done?"

☐ **Black and white thinking:** This is the tendency to place all experiences in one of two opposite categories. You view situations as either black or white and you do not see the shades of grey in between. For example, things are either "good or bad," "terrible or terrific," "a complete success or a total failure." In describing yourself, you tend to select the extreme negative category. For example, you think "I made a mistake on that … the whole job is ruined."

☐ **The fortune teller:** You anticipate that things will turn out badly, and you feel convinced that your prediction is an already established fact. For example, "I'll fail that exam."

☐ **Emotional reasoning:** You assume that your negative emotions necessarily reflect the way things really are. For example, "I feel bad, so things must be going badly," "I feel depressed, therefore my marriage is not working out."

☐ **"Should" statements:** You try to motivate yourself with shoulds, musts, and oughts. If you find yourself unable to do something, you then feel guilty and demoralized. For example, "I should be able to understand this the first time I read it."

☐ **Labeling/judgmental focus:** You assign global negative traits to yourself and others. For example, "He's a total loser," "I'm stupid." You view yourself, others, and events in terms of evaluations as good–bad, superior–inferior, rather than simply describing, accepting, or understanding. You continually find that you and others fall short of your high expectations.

☐ **Dismissing the evidence:** You reject any evidence or arguments that contradict your negative thoughts. For example, when you have the thought "I'm unlovable," you reject as irrelevant any evidence that people like you, "That's not the real issue; there are deeper problems and other factors." Consequently, your thought cannot be refuted.

> These all sound familiar to me!

Everyone engages in unhelpful thinking at times, especially when they are under stress. However, these unhelpful thinking patterns can occur very frequently when people have GAD.

If we boil these thinking errors right down, we can see that they all overestimate how bad situations truly are and underestimate your ability to cope. We need to learn to shift unhelpful thinking.

Challenging worry thinking

Thought challenging is about becoming more flexible in the way you think. We are not aiming for positive thinking; we want you to develop thinking that is *realistic, helpful, and constructive.* Thought challenging involves four steps.

Step 1: Identify the situation and recognize your thoughts

When you start to feel distressed, it is important to stop and ask yourself what is going on. Ask yourself, "What am I worried will happen or is happening?" or "What is the worst that could happen?".

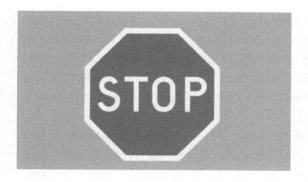

Step 2: Test whether your thoughts are realistic

Think of yourself as a scientist. You are trying to find out if there is convincing evidence that your worries are realistic or accurate. The best way to do this is to ask questions. You will not need to answer every question; just try some out and see which ones work best for you. Here is a list of questions you can try:

- *Put it under the microscope*: What is the evidence that these thoughts are not 100% true? What are the *facts*?
- *Rewind*: What happened last time I worried about this? How did I cope?
- *Be a detective*: Am I jumping to conclusions? Am I making any errors in my thinking? What is an alternative explanation? What is most likely to happen?
- *Try a different perspective*: Would everyone think this way? What would I say to a friend if they were in this situation? Are there any positives or opportunities in this situation?
- *Leave judging to a judge*: Am I being overly critical? Is it helpful to think like this?
- *Fast forward*: Will this situation still be bad in a week/month/year? Even if the worst happens, how could I cope?

Step 3: Shift thoughts to be more realistic and helpful

After you have challenged the worry thoughts, summarize what you have come up with. Consider developing a more realistic and helpful way to look at the situation.

Step 4: Conduct an experiment

It is difficult to think in new ways. New thoughts do not *feel* convincing, even if they seem more logical. Conducting worry experiments is very helpful here. Like many things in life, "seeing is believing" and it is not until you actually *do things differently* that you can think in different ways.

The best experiments are ones that are *specific*. Try to think what would be a clear and direct test of your worries. When scientists conduct experiments, they *repeat* them and *record* their results and see if their predictions came true or not. So, after challenging your worries in the first three steps, carry out an experiment to see if your fears actually come true or not.

> The four steps in thought challenging are recorded on a "thought-challenging record." I've shown you one of my examples (see Table 6.5).
>
> This was a really hard skill for me—my challenges did not seem very convincing, but I remembered that that wasn't the point. The point was to be more flexible in the way I viewed situations... so I just kept trying.
>
> Writing my worries down was very good. It gave me some perspective and helped me get some distance from the worry.

> It helps to "stick to the facts" and "play the odds." I need to put things into perspective and focus on what is most likely to happen, rather than assuming things will be a disaster. However, there's always something new to worry about. Just when I've dealt with one worry—another pops up! I worry I'll be doing these records forever! Is that true?

Good question Liz! That is very common. This skill is about helping you respond to anxiety-producing situations in a different way. One response is to worry—that is what you normally do. Thought challenging encourages you to stop and reflect on how accurate your fears are and to practice letting them go if they are not realistic. Over time, we expect that this skill will become more automatic and that you can let go of worries more rapidly—even if they are new worries.

Table 6.5 Liz's thought challenging record (There is a blank record for you in the back of this manual; see Form 6.5)

Identify the situation and recognize your thoughts	Test whether your thoughts are realistic (Use the list of questions)	Shift thoughts to be more realistic and helpful
Situation: Finishing work report—deadline is tomorrow **Thoughts:** This report must be perfect If the report has mistakes in it, my boss is bound to pick them up She will notice all the other mistakes I make She will think I am incompetent and that I am a fraud I will get fired I will not find a new job We will not be able to pay our mortgage We will be destitute	Sometimes when I make mistakes, no one notices them. Sometimes my boss does notice them and corrects them. She has not said I am not good at my job—in fact, my last performance review was positive. My boss makes mistakes, and I do not think she is a fraud or incompetent. Everyone makes mistakes. Other people at work learn from their mistakes; they do not get fired for them (unless they are really big). I have been retrenched before, but that was not because of mistakes I had made—the company was restructuring. I did eventually find a new job, and we were able to pay our mortgage by reorganizing the loan. Even if we lost our house, we could live with my parents or my in-laws until we sorted out our finances. **Unhelpful thinking patterns:** Catastrophizing, black and white thinking, the fortune teller, jumping to conclusions, mind reading	I do not like making mistakes, I never have, but pretty much everyone I know makes mistakes. It is not likely that I will get fired for making everyday mistakes in my report. My boss thinks I am a good worker. Even if I get fired, we will cope. **What experiment could I conduct to test this worry out?** Leave a small mistake in my report. Ask my boss what she thought of the report. **What happened?** My boss noticed the mistake and corrected it. She also noticed a few other mistakes I did not know were there. However, she said it was a good report.

The last step in thought challenging, worry experiments, really helped me see that most of the things I worry about don't happen. Here are some of the things I did . . . (see Table 6.6)

Table 6.6 Worry experiments

Worry	Experiment	Outcome
This headache will never end. What if it is a brain tumor!	Do not rush to the doctor. Take some paracetamol and get on with my day.	My headache went away. I coped without my doctor!
If I say no to Eddy, he will think I do not like him.	Next time Eddy asks to have coffee, tell him I cannot make it this time. See if he is upset and does not ask me again.	He was a bit disappointed but he asked another time.
If I drive to a new place, I will get lost and something terrible will happen (car break down/get attacked/ have a panic attack).	Pick a quiet afternoon and drive to a suburb I have never been to before. Just see what happens.	I did get lost but used a map to find my way home. Nothing bad happened; I was just a bit tired and tense.
What if something bad happens to my kids and they cannot contact me? How irresponsible … they could die!	Turn mobile phone off during work meetings and when driving.	I had a few missed calls—not from the kids. Nothing bad happened.

A special note about coping with doubt and uncertainty

Both thought challenging and worry experiments involve tolerating doubt and uncertainty. This happens whenever we try to think or act differently. Often, people feel that they cannot allow themselves to feel uncertain because they worry they will not cope or that something bad will happen. You may have beliefs like:

◆ A small unforeseen event can spoil everything, even with the best planning.

◆ I cannot take chances, even if it is highly unlikely that something bad might happen.

+ When I am uncertain, I cannot function very well.
+ The smallest doubt can stop me from acting.
+ I cannot stand being taken by surprise.

You can challenge these beliefs using your thought challenging record. The fact is that we frequently tolerate doubt and uncertainty in our lives—we just may not realize it! Every week, you may be taking sensible and calculated risks. The following is a brief list of activities that people commonly engage in; they all involve some degree of uncertainty. Tick the ones you have done in your life:

☐ Drive a car or be a passenger in a car

☐ Take public transport

☐ Fly in an airplane

☐ Eat in a restaurant

☐ Go to the city in the night-time

☐ Drink alcohol or smoke cigarettes

☐ Visit a sick friend or walk through a hospital

☐ Go overseas

☐ Ride a bike or horse

☐ Pat a dog or own a pet

☐ Go on a date (or ask someone out on a date)

☐ Have an operation, give birth, or take medications

☐ Swim in the ocean

☐ Give your opinion

☐ Buy or rent a property or invest in shares

☐ Attend school, college, or university

☐ Go to the gym or play sport

☐ Go out in the hot sun

☐ Eat food close to its "use by" date

☐ Cross the street

☐ Turn on the hot water tap

☐ Maintain a friendship/ relationship

> I've actually done all of these! I didn't think of these things as taking a risk.

Most people do these things because they have learned to tolerate the uncertainty and believe the benefits of doing the activity outweigh the risks involved.

> Maybe it is not even possible to avoid uncertainty? You can't always be in control and know what is going to happen! There are lots of things I try to control—my health, the housework, what other people think of me, my work schedule—but really, when I think about it, unexpected things often happen that throw my plans out. I need to be more flexible and be less concerned about unexpected things.

That's right Liz. We all have some control in our lives, but lots of things happen outside of our control. Our efforts to have complete control and avoid all uncertainty are doomed to failure. Worry can give us an illusion of control and predictability; it can feel like it reduces our doubt and uncertainty. Really, however, we often worry about things that never happen. We need to accept uncertainty in life and let go of our attempts to control things unnecessarily. So, we would encourage you to challenge your worries about uncertainty and control, and conduct lots experiments!

If you are concerned that you will not be able to cope, try to break the problem down into more manageable pieces. Also, take a few minutes to think back over your life and consider some of the really challenging situations you have faced. How did you cope? How do other people cope when they are faced with similar challenges? Perhaps you are better able to cope with distress and uncertainty than you are giving yourself credit for?

Coping with problems

> *Some of my worries are realistic—I really do have problems with this woman at work and I really do have debt!*
>
> *I have been 'catastrophizing' about these situations, and the thought challenging has helped me reduce this—but I still have to deal with these problems…*

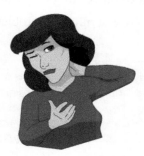

Many people with GAD worry about daily problems and sources of stress (e.g., budgeting, managing family or work conflicts and duties, completing studies, dealing with unemployment or sickness). These problems *are happening right now* and need to be solved.

However, you may also worry about things that are *not* happening at the moment; they are hypothetical problems that may or may not happen at some point in the future. For example, Penny is medically well but worries about her health. She worries about her lack of exercise (current problem) and also about dying from diabetes complications (hypothetical problem).

How can I tell the difference between a current problem and a hypothetical problem?

It may be helpful to do a thought challenging record and truthfully ask yourself:

- Is my problem very likely to happen?

- Is it happening right now or will it happen very soon?

- Can I do anything about it?

- Would other people in my life agree with my answers to these questions?

If the answer is yes to these questions, then you are probably facing a current problem.

Often, people with GAD have a good idea about how to solve problems, but worries about solving them can get in the way. These worries can include thoughts like:

- My problems are insurmountable.
- I am no good at solving problems.
- My problems are too confronting—I should just avoid them.
- I am not capable of overcoming my problems.

> Thoughts like these stop me from facing my problems. I tend to procrastinate and criticize myself instead . . . but that just makes everything worse!
>
> I did a thought-challenging record on these thoughts and when I really looked at the evidence, I discovered that I have actually managed to overcome many problems in my life. Looking back, I also realized that dealing with my problems gave me lots of chances to learn new things.

Structured problem solving

A great way to experiment with worries about not being able to solve problems is to use the "structured problem-solving technique." It is a five-step process that can be used to combat problems that are happening right now and that you are avoiding dealing with. It is another way of responding to difficulties besides worry. It is important to give your full attention to the technique and allow yourself enough time to work through it properly and to write your solutions down.

Step 1: Identify the problem or goal

Gaining a clear definition of the problem or goal is a vital step in problem solving. You need to focus on the main problem and avoid getting side tracked by minor details and other issues.

When you are defining your problem:

- Write a list of all your current problems and pick one to focus on. Only consider one problem or goal at a time. If other problems arise, leave them for another time.
- Make the problem as specific as possible. This may involve breaking it down into a smaller part. For example, the problem "I'm broke" could

be broken down to the specific problem "My credit card repayment is due next Wednesday and I am unable to pay it" or "I want to get fit" could be "I want to exercise three times a week."

Step 2: Generate solutions

Now think of as many solutions as possible. Do not try to work out what the best or perfect solution is; just list any ideas that come to mind—including those which may not be useful or sound silly. Use your imagination! Do not evaluate the solutions; just write them down.

Step 3: Evaluate the solutions and choose one

Briefly consider the advantages and disadvantages of each solution. There is no need to write these points down in detail but just quickly run through the list of solutions, noting the strengths and weaknesses of each. Remember, no solution will be perfect and provide 100% certainty!

Next, choose the solution (or combination of solutions) which will begin to solve the problem. Choose something that you can implement straightaway. It may not be ideal or solve the problem immediately, but it may make a difference and help you work out what to do next.

Step 4: Plan

Write out a brief step-by-step plan of action. It will help you carry out your solution. Consider:

* Do I have what I need (e.g., time, skills, equipment) or do I need to arrange them?
* Do I have the co-operation of others who are involved in the plan?
* When will I carry out my plan?

Step 5: Review

After implementing your plan, think about what you have achieved and what the next step is. Most problems are not completely solved after the first round of structured problem solving and sometimes things even get worse. This review activity is a good chance to ask:

* What went right? What went wrong?
* What could I do next time?
* Who can help me with this problem?

Remember to still encourage yourself and acknowledge your efforts, even if things did not work out as you would have liked.

Table 6.7 is an example of this five-step process as completed by Liz. There is a blank problem-solving worksheet at the back of this manual

Table 6.7 Liz's structured problem-solving worksheet (A blank worksheet is at the back of this manual; see Form 6.6)

Step 1: What is the problem/ goal? Carefully think about what the problem is —the more narrowly you can define it, the better.	I do not have enough money to pay my credit card bill.
Step 2: List all possible solutions Put down all ideas, even bad ones!	1. Buy lottery tickets 2. Ask Dad for a loan 3. Ring the bank and ask for more time to pay 4. Get another job 5. Ring a helpline for people with debt problems 6. Do nothing and hope the problem goes away
Step 3: Evaluate each possible solution *Quickly* go down the list of solutions and consider the advantages and disadvantages of each.	1. Easy, but probably will not win and tickets cost money. 2. Quick, but Dad does not have any money to spare. Plus, he would be angry with me. 3. They could give me an extension, which would be good. However, I am embarrassed. I am worried they will yell at me. 4. Would give me more money over the long term, but I do not have enough energy right now. 5. Free, quick, could be helpful, but I am embarrassed and ashamed. 6. Easiest option, but problem will only get worse. Will not solve anything.
Choose a solution Pick the best solution; try to pick one that you can start to work on straight away.	Ring debt helpline
Step 4: Plan how to carry out the solution Plan out, step by step, what you will do.	1. Look up number in the phone book.To be done: 5 pm today 2. Do thought challenging record about making the call.To be done: Saturday 10 am 3. Make the call.To be done: Monday 9 am 4. Review progress: Monday 6 pm
Step 5: Review progress Focus on the things you have achieved and be pleased with any progress you have made.	I made the call and the person I spoke to was really nice. She made an appointment for me to see a financial counselor who will help me.
Consider what needs to be done next	I need to go to the appointment. I am very nervous about it, so I will do a thought challenging record first.

for you. Here are some extra tips for your structured problem solving. Remember:

- Problems are a normal part of life—try to think of them as challenges to overcome rather than impossible or dangerous.

- Do not forget to search for any positive opportunities that may go along with your problem. Is this problem giving you a chance to learn new skills, build your coping capacity, develop your relationships, or find out more about yourself and your values?

- If you feel overwhelmed, a friend may be able to help you use the problem-solving technique.

- When solving a problem, do not get caught up in small detail—stay focused on the main problem.

- Avoid avoiding—problems grow when you do not deal with them.

- Press on even if you feel unsure and anxious. Try to tolerate uncomfortable feelings and implement your solution as best you can.

- There may be some problems that you cannot resolve because they are out of your control (e.g., changing another person's beliefs or behaviors). In these cases, the problem-solving technique may help you develop a plan of how you can cope with the situation.

Summary

During Section 4, we explored how worrying thoughts contribute to GAD. The skills we introduced you to include:

- Recognizing unhelpful thinking styles (e.g., catastrophizing, black and white thinking)

- Thought challenging for worries

  - that pop up in everyday situations
  - about uncertainty and coping
  - about dealing with problems

- Worry experiments

- Structured problem solving for problems you are facing at the moment

Mastering these skills takes lots of practice and effort. Please do not feel discouraged if you find these skills difficult to begin with—the more you use them, the easier they become.

Remember, you may have had difficulties with anxiety and worry for years, so do not expect that you will be able to change your worry habits straightaway. Instead, try to encourage yourself for the effort you are putting in. We know these skills can help, so do not give up!

Over the next few weeks, aim to use these skills as often as possible. It may also be helpful to continue using your controlled breathing, relaxation, and exercise skills from the previous section. Good luck and we will see you again soon!

Section 5: ADVANCED SKILLS FOR MANAGING WORRY THOUGHTS

In this section, we take a closer look at the beliefs you may have about your worry. Allow yourself several weeks to work through this section and complete all the exercises.

Beliefs about worry tend to be negative (e.g., "my worry is making me sick") or positive (e.g., "my worry helps me get things done"). Positive beliefs motivate you to worry, while negative beliefs are likely to make you worry about the worry. These beliefs keep the worry cycle going.

> I'm not sure what my beliefs about worry are!

Look back at Section 2 where you identified beliefs about worry. You can also list the particular advantages and disadvantages that worry has for you. Have a look at Liz's list (see Table 6.8) and then add your own ideas to it—try to be specific.

Negative beliefs about worry

Let us start with the negative beliefs. Most negative beliefs revolve around the notion that worry is uncontrollable or that it is dangerous in some way. It is important to stop and evaluate how accurate these beliefs truly are. If they are not very true, then you may not need to be so worried about your worrying!

We can use the same process we did earlier by questioning the evidence for your beliefs and then conducting some experiments. Step 1 is to identify the belief you want to challenge.

Table 6.8 Liz's disadvantages and advantages of worry

Liz's disadvantages of worry	Liz's advantages of worry
My worry is uncontrollable	Worry helps me avoid mistakes in my reports
Worry stops me enjoying things (like family outings)	I will not get to places on time without worrying
My worry will never end	If anything bad happens, I will be prepared/not taken by surprise
Worry makes me irritable and tense	My family is safe, happy, and healthy because I worry about them
I'll get sick or go crazy from worrying too much	
Your disadvantages of worry	**Your advantages of worry**

I'll start with my top one—"my worry is uncontrollable."

Okay Liz. Now before we go any further, we need to work out exactly what you mean because "uncontrollable worry" may mean different things to different people. So, it often helps to think about what "uncontrollable worry" would actually look like.

What do you mean?

Let us make some predictions based on this belief that your worry is uncontrollable. Let us say your worry truly is uncontrollable. Now, imagine you were worrying a great deal—as much as possible. What would happen?

> I would be out of control. . . .

And what would that look like … if we took a video of you being "out of control?" What would we see?

> I would be crying, maybe screaming. I couldn't do anything—I wouldn't be able to think about anything else, just my worry. My worry would last forever. I wouldn't be able to get out of bed or do things around the house. I think people would look at me as if I were crazy or stupid. Eventually, my husband would call the doctor and I would hospitalized.

Okay, now we have a very clear picture of what this belief means to you. Let us question how realistic this scenario is. Here are some questions, and we will use a new sort of thought- challenging record:

- *Rewind*: Has this ever happened before? When these difficult things did happen, how did you cope?
- *Glass half full*: Have there been times when your worry was under control (e.g., you were distracted by something, too busy to worry, able to postpone the worry, or the worry got interrupted)?
- *Be a detective*: Have there been times when your worry was not dangerous or harmful (e.g., you worried and did not get sick, go crazy, get in trouble, hurt others)?
- *Fast forward*: Does your worry eventually die down? What happens then?
- *Walk in someone else's shoes*: Do most people believe worry is uncontrollable or dangerous? Some peoples' jobs are very stressful (e.g., paramedics, police, soldiers), does worry hurt them all the time?
- *Weigh it up*: Besides the worry, are there other reasons that difficult things have happened (e.g., other than worry, what other factors lead to getting sick, being unemployed, going to hospital, relationship breakdowns)?

Using these questions, Liz challenged her belief that "my worry is uncontrollable." Take a look at what she came up with on her thought-challenging record (see Tables 6.9 and 6.10). (Note that a blank record for you can be found at the end of this manual; see Form 6.7.)

Table 6.9 Liz challenges a negative belief about worry (example 1)

Identify the negative belief about your worry	Test whether your belief is realistic (use your list of questions)	Change the belief to be more realistic and helpful
Belief: My worry is uncontrollable	**Has this ever happened?** Not to that extent, but one time I was very worried and depressed and I wanted to stay in bed forever, but I did not. I made myself get up. I was crying a bit, but not screaming. It lasted about 3 weeks, but I did not go to hospital.	My worry feels uncontrollable, but it is not. Even at my worst, I have not lost control of myself. My worry does not go on forever, and a lot of times I eventually get distracted by something else and my worry gets forgotten. Sometimes I am even too busy to worry—so I must have some control over it.
Clarify what this belief means to you. If this belief was true, and you worried a lot, what do you fear would happen?	Weighing it up, this was depression as well as the worry. I had been having problems at work and with my husband. I was not looking after myself and my best friend was overseas ... all these things contributed, it was not just the worry.	**What experiment could you conduct to test this belief?**
I would be crying and screaming. I could not do anything—stuck in bed all day and night. Could not think of anything besides my worry. It would never stop. People would think I was crazy. I would be hospitalized.	**How did I cope?** People did not think I was crazy—my doctor was actually kind and I started some medication which helped. I tried to get back to my normal routine, and spent more time with my good friends. It did not last forever—I did get better.	I will see if I can postpone my worry. If I can do this—even just a little bit—it will show that the worry is not uncontrollable. Here are my steps: 1. Pick a worry "I'll get fired." 2. When that worry pops up, see if I can postpone it. Tell myself "I will worry about this later." Then I will get back to work as best I can. 3. Pick a time to worry about it later. My "worry time" is at 3.30 pm—when I have afternoon tea. 4. When my worry time arrives, I will worry about getting fired for 5 minutes.
	Now when I think about it, I am able to control my worry—at least some of the time. I tend to forget my worry when I am distracted by something, especially when I am busy at work or with my friends.	**What happened?**
	My worry does eventually fade away. It has never gone on forever. Things change in my life, and I move on from a worry—sometimes things feel different after a sleep. Worries are temporary.	I did this every day for a week. I could postpone the worry on four days. Most days when my worry time came around, I did not feel the need to worry—it felt a bit silly really. I guess I have more control over the worry than I thought.
	I do not know, but I suspect most people do not think worry is uncontrollable. Everyone worries about something. If worry were really uncontrollable, everyone would be very stressed out, and that is not the case.	

Tip!

To help postpone worries, you could try keeping busy, doing some exercise, calling a friend, or trying the strategies outlined in the section 'Letting go of worries'. Some people write down the worry in a journal and then get back to it later.

Table 6.10 Liz challenges a negative belief about worry (example 2)

Identify the negative belief about your worry	Test whether your belief is realistic (use the list of questions)	Change the belief to be more realistic and helpful
Belief: I will get sick or go crazy from worrying too much	**Has this ever happened?** No! I have been a worrier my whole life, and never had a heart attack, fainted, or gone crazy. I feel like I will, but I do not.	Worry feels really bad, but it is not dangerous—it does not send me crazy or make me seriously ill. The fight/flight response is supposed to help protect me, so it does not make sense that it is dangerous.
Clarify what this belief means to you. If this belief was true, and you worried a lot, what do you fear would happen?	I do get more colds than most of my friends, which could be the worry, but it could also be that I work in a busy office with lots of people. Plus, the kids often bring colds home from school. Plus, there have been plenty of times in my life that I have been sick even though I have not been particularly worried.	**What experiment could you conduct to test this belief?** I could see if worry makes me go crazy or gives me a cold by purposefully worrying for 5 minutes. Here are my steps:
I would have a heart attack or faint. I might go crazy—lose control of my body or lose touch with reality.	**How could I cope?** I guess I would go to hospital and get treatment if I had a heart attack, got cancer, or became psychotic. If my worry is lowering my immune system, I need to take better care of myself—eat well, exercise, and take time off.	1. Pick a couple of worries. 2. Set aside a time to really worry about these things for a full 5 minutes. 3. At the specified time, write out and think through all the worries and try to really lose control.
I also believe my worry is slowly wearing down my immune system—so I will get frequent colds/flu, and eventually get cancer.	Weigh it up—heart attacks usually happen in people with heart disease, which is partly related to genes and unhealthy lifestyle—eating unhealthy food, not exercising, drinking, smoking. This is also the case with cancer. When I looked up the risk factors for cancer, they did not mention worry!	**What happened?** Nothing! I did this for 3 days in a row, but I did not get a cold. I felt very upset on the first day, but I did not lose control of my body or my mind. I felt a bit silly by the third day.
	Two of my friends have cancer—one is anxious like me, but the other one is not. Plus, people with stressful jobs do not have heart attacks all the time or get cancer, or become psychotic more than people with less stressful jobs.	

> Being able to postpone my worry was a real surprise to me. I decided to use "worry time" every day. When I noticed myself worrying during the day, I "saved it up" until my scheduled worry time—usually the same time and place every day. At that time, I focused on my worries for about 15 minutes each day. Lots of times, I found I didn't feel like worrying, but when I did, I made sure I had planned a good activity to take my mind off the worry after my 15 minutes were up.

Now, let us take a look at the other type of negative belief most people with GAD have— that "my worry is dangerous/harmful" in some way. Here is Liz's thought-challenging record. (A blank record for you can be found at the end of this manual; see Form 6.7.)

Tips!

Fainting fears? In order to faint, your blood pressure needs to drop. However, when you are anxious, your blood pressure actually rises—it is part of the fight/flight response. Some people do faint in specific situations (e.g., seeing blood, getting very hot) but this is related to a specific vasovagal response.

Heart attack fears? How is the heart restarted when it has stopped beating? Doctors administer adrenaline. Adrenaline gets pumped through your heart when you are anxious. Anxiety does not give you heart attacks—otherwise everyone would have heart attacks.

Diseases? Worry that your worry will cause a specific disease? Check out the facts by asking your doctor about the known causes of the disease that you worry about.

We have got a list of experiments you can try in order to test negative beliefs about worry (see Table 6.11).

> When I questioned and experimented with my beliefs, I found that my negative beliefs weren't 100% true. I was exaggerating how bad worry is—worry may not be a good thing—and I don't think it is dangerous or uncontrollable now.
>
> Then I started to think, if my worry is not out of control or harmful, maybe I don't need to put pressure on myself to control my worry. I don't need to push the worries away or criticize myself when a worry pops into my head. I don't need to reassure myself or tell myself to think positively.

Table 6.11 Experiments to test negative beliefs about worry

Negative beliefs about worry	Possible experiment
Strong people do not worry My worry means I am weak	Conduct a brief survey of people you know—some who you consider "strong" and some you consider "weak." Ask if and when they worry, and what they worry about. Alternatively, survey "strong" people and make the survey anonymous. *Note*: you do not need to say why you are doing the survey or you can give a reason that protects your privacy.
My worry harms others	Define what you mean by "harm" (physical, emotional, or social). Pick a few people to worry about. Set aside a time to intensely worry about these people for a full 5 minutes. At the specified time, start worrying. Assess if your worry has harmed any of the people you worried about. *Extra tip*: Some people will alternate days they do and do not do the 5-minute worry session. If the belief is true, on the non-worry days, there should be no or less harm to the people worried about.
My worry stops me enjoying things	Pick an easily repeated activity that you enjoy (e.g., movies, swimming, socializing). Before you engage in the activity, spend 5 minutes worrying about something. Then engage in the activity as fully as you can. Notice if you are able to enjoy the activity at all. The next time you do the activity, do not do the 5-minute worry session. Compare the two experiences and notice if the worry session had a big impact on your enjoyment levels.
People will reject me if they know I worry	List the people you think will reject you. Pick one that you know well and who is a good listener. During a conversation, ask them if they worry about things in their life and what they think about people who worry. If you are comfortable, let them know that you often worry about things. *Tip*: You may want to repeat this experiment with other people.

That is right Liz. In fact, a lot of people find that the more they try to avoid, suppress, or control their worry, the worse it gets. A better option is to learn to let worries go—we will get to that soon—but it is hard to let something go if you feel it is helping you cope.

Positive beliefs about worry

People with GAD often believe that there are benefits to worrying. Look back to the beginning of this section where you listed the advantages of worrying, as well as to the beliefs you selected in Section 2 about how worry may be helpful to you. If these benefits were false, you would be less motivated to worry.

> So I guess the first step is to challenge these beliefs, and then do some experiments? Check out Table 6.12.

Absolutely! Here is a list of questions to help you challenge these beliefs (a blank thought- challenging record for you can be found at the end of this manual; see Form 6.8):

- *Be a detective*: Has this happened before? Are there times when you did not worry and things have been OK?

- *Dissect it*: How exactly does worry prevent bad things from happening or prepare you?

- *Glass is half empty*: Have there been times when your worry has not helped you (e.g., helped you cope, solve problems, prepare you, motivate you, or take care of your health)?

- *Weigh it up*: Besides worry, what else helps you cope with problems? Consider:

  - your determination, intelligence, experience, thoughtfulness, resourcefulness, communication skills

  - your ability to work hard, be organized, get help from others

  - the passage of time

  - money

  - coincidence/good luck

- *Put it in perspective*: Besides worry, what else shows you care about others? Would you rather have your loved ones worry about you or show they care about you in other ways? Would you recommend worrying to your loved ones to help them deal with their difficulties?

- *Mismatch*: How can worry be helpful if it is also distressing, excessive, and negatively interferes in your life?

- *Walk in someone else's shoes*: When difficult things happen to people you care about (e.g., getting very sick, being in an accident, losing their job), is it because they did not worry enough about these things, or are there other reasons why people experience hardships?

Table 6.12 Liz challenges a positive belief about worry

Identify the positive belief about your worry	Test whether your belief is realistic (use the list of questions)	Change the belief to be more realistic and helpful
Belief: Worry prepares me—it stops me being taken by surprise. **Clarify what this belief means to you.** If this belief was true, and you worried a lot, what would happen? Nothing unexpected would happen. I would be in control all the time. When problems arise, I would know how to deal with them because I would have worried about them ahead of time.	**Has this happened before?** I worry about what to say in work meetings and sometimes I can anticipate the questions I will be asked. However, most of the time, I need to think on my feet. If I am really honest, I rely on my experience and hard work to get me through (not worry). Although I am not very good at asking for help, I know people are there for me when I need it. Things rarely go 100% according to plan—unexpected things pop up all the time at work and with the kids. Often things happen that I have not worried about, like unexpected visitors or new deadlines. Often worry does not help me be prepared because I end up procrastinating and seeking reassurance rather than getting on with the task. Most of the things I worry about do not happen, so I am not really preparing myself for dealing with real problems. When I think of people in my life who seem most "in control" and "on top of things," I do not think it is because they worry. I think it is because they are confident, smart, level-headed, and hard-working.	Worry gives me the feeling of being prepared and in control, but it is more likely that I can manage when unexpected things happen because—as my boss says—I am a capable person. **What experiment could you conduct to test this belief?** I will see how prepared worry really makes me. I will ask friends over to dinner. The first time, I will worry ahead of time and try to control anything unexpected. The second time I have friends over, I will avoid worrying and just work it out on the day. If worry prepares me, then the first dinner should be trouble-free with no surprises. The second dinner will not be like that. **What happened?** I was a lot more stressed before the first dinner—trying to get everything perfect. In the end, both dinners were enjoyable once they got going. Unexpected things happened on both occasions—people running late and Jenny announcing she is pregnant. However, I coped just fine—we just made do. My worry did not really prepare me because pretty much everything I thought would go wrong, did not happen. The worry just added extra pressure.

Table 6.13 includes some sample experiments for positive beliefs about worry.

Table 6.13 Experiments to test positive beliefs about worry

Positive beliefs about worry	Possible experiment
My worries are realistic and likely to happen	Pick an oncoming event that you are worried about. Spend 15 minutes writing down, in lots of detail, all the things you worry will happen—be very specific! After the event, write down (again in detail) what actually happened. Now, compare the two papers and see how accurate the worry truly was. Repeat this experiment on several occasions. Ask yourself, if your worry is not accurate, how can it be truly helpful?
Worry protects those I care about	Pick a person to worry about. On day one, increase your worry about their welfare (e.g., purposefully worry for 5 minutes about something bad happening to them). On day two, avoid this worry session. On day three, engage in the worry session. On day four, avoid the worry session. Continue this until you have enough information about whether your loved one experiences less hardship on worry days and more hardship on non-worry days. *Note:* Do not tell the person you are worrying about them, or change your behavior towards them—just worry more or less about them.
Worry stops bad things from happening	Pick a bad event that happens regularly (e.g., crimes reported on the news, heavy traffic, or political scandals). On day one, increase your worry about this event in order to prevent it (e.g., purposefully worry for 5 minutes about something bad happening). On day two, avoid this worry session. On day three, engage in the worry session. On day four, avoid the worry session. Continue this until you have enough information about whether your worry has stopped the bad thing from happening. *Note:* Remember to take into account the additional causes of bad events (e.g., the time of year, the weather).
Worry helps me solve problems	Compare worrying to structured problem solving. Pick a problem you would like to solve. First, use worry to address it. Write out the problem and then describe the worst outcome possible (i.e., what you worry will happen—allow your mind to run through all the "what ifs ..."). The following day, use the structure problem-solving technique to address the problem. Compare how helpful each strategy was at finding solutions to the problem.
Worry helps me be more efficient	Select an activity, your efficiency at which you think is improved by worry. The next time you do the task, spend 5 minutes worrying about it beforehand. Make a note of how efficient you were on a scale of 0–10. The next time you do the task, avoid worrying and just do the task straightaway. Again, rate your efficiency out of 10. Repeat these two procedures until you have a clear picture of whether the worry significantly increases your efficiency (e.g., by more than five points).

In summary ...

A lot of experiments with worry are about increasing or decreasing the amount of worry that you engage in and seeing what happens as a result. If our negative beliefs are true, we would expect bad things to happen (e.g., getting sick, running mad, never ending worry). If our positive beliefs are true, we would expect good things to happen (e.g., feeling calm and in control of everything, increased productivity, great relationships). Both sets of beliefs cannot be completely true—but both can be false!

> I had never actually thought about my beliefs about worry. I've always relied on worry to help me cope, but now I see there are other ways of coping. Now I am beginning to understand that my worry is not dangerous, and it is not helpful either. So what do I do when worries pop into my head?

Letting go of worries

Our minds have thousands of thoughts every day. Is it possible to listen and respond to all of them? If we did, would anyone get anything done? The fact is that we all learn to "let go" of many of our thoughts. Sometimes we get back to them later, sometimes not.

Anxious thoughts and feelings grab our attention and demand to be taken seriously. This is part of the fight/flight response; worries seem very important because they appear to alert us to potential threats and dangers. However, in GAD, worries are false alarms and constantly responding to them is unhelpful.

Imagine if your worries were internet pop-ups. If you clicked on every one and thoroughly investigated them before dismissing them, you would struggle to finish your work and would become increasingly agitated. We may not be able to stop pop-ups, but we do not need to click on them. You cannot stop thoughts coming into your mind, but you can learn to just let them come and go without constantly responding to them.

> So, how do I do that? How do I let go of worries?

"Letting go" can be a tricky skill to get your head around. We want to avoid responding to worries in unhelpful ways, like seeking reassurance, arguing with the worry, or worrying about the worry. Instead, we want to get back to the task at hand. There following are three steps to do that.

Step 1. Stop and watch

Notice that you are worried. You need to be aware of what you are doing in order to let go of doing it! The first signs may be physical sensations, like tense shoulders. Now, just watch the worry—the thoughts, physical sensations, the urges to do things like avoid or seek reassurance. Try not to judge your experiences by evaluating them as good or bad, rational or irrational, right or wrong.

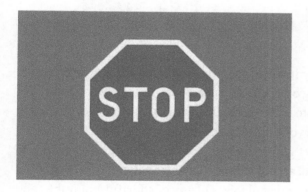

Step 2. Choose to let the worry go

You can decide to keep worrying or to let it go. It may take practice, but you can choose what you focus on. Some people find it helpful to talk themselves through the decision (e.g., saying to yourself "let it go," "that's a worry thought—I don't want to focus on that now," "I can't do anything about this now; I need to get on with other things"). Others use mental imagery, such as seeing their worries as clouds or leaves passing by on the wind, or imagining their worries are on an express train that is traveling past them.

Step 3. Focus on the present

Do you spend a lot of time worrying about the future and analyzing the past?

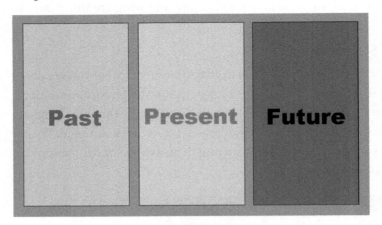

Letting go of worry involves turning your mind back to the present moment and focusing on what you are actually doing. This may be typing an email, talking to a friend, feeding the dog … whatever the task at hand is, that is where your mind needs to be.

It can be hard to let go of worry if you do not have other things to occupy your mind. So, an important part of managing worry is finding ways to ensure that your day involves plenty of effortful, enjoyable, and meaningful activities. Some people schedule in activities (like reading a magazine or doing some exercise) when they know they will have too much time on their hands and they are likely to start worrying. It is up to you to find out what works best for you.

> Sometimes it hard to focus back on what I am doing. Are there any strategies that can help me?

If you are having trouble letting thoughts just come and go, some people find it helpful to use a simple and brief "circuit breaker" type activity to help them disengage from the worry and return to the present. Some examples include:

- Focus on your breathing.
- Do some brief relaxation.
- Focus on where you are—name five things you can see and hear, then four new things you can see and hear, then three etc ...
- Coach yourself (e.g., "It's ok, it's worry. It's normal to feel anxious. This will pass. You can do this. Just try to let go of the worry".)

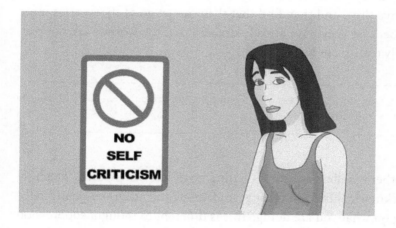

These strategies may help you get a little distance or space from the worry, so it is easier to focus back on the present activity or task at hand.

> When I let go of my worries, they often pop back in again. My mind seems to wander all over the place ...

This is completely normal—that is just what minds do. Just keep turning your mind back to what you are doing and try to avoid criticizing yourself and becoming too frustrated. Just let time pass and let the worries come and go. It is not your job to get rid of worry thoughts; it is your job to return your mind to the present.

> But I thought I was supposed to challenge my worry thoughts? I'm confused—when do I let worries go and when do I challenge them?

Good question! The two skills complement each other and are both aimed at helping you disengage from unhelpful worry and get on with what you are doing. Challenging worries takes time, whereas letting go of them is often much quicker, which makes it practical to use frequently throughout the day. Most people challenge their worries when they have time, and then find that they can let go of the worries more easily because they have already decided that the worries are not particularly realistic or helpful.

> Is letting go of worries like distraction or thought suppression? Aren't these unhelpful thought-control strategies?

Another excellent question! Letting go of worries involves watching and acknowledging the feelings and thoughts, and then gently refocusing on what you are doing. This is different to thought suppression where we are trying to purposefully push worries away because we are afraid they are dangerous. The emphasis in this skill is on a positive action—returning your mind to the present and getting on with your day. It is not an avoidance-based strategy, which is what trying not to think something is.

Distraction is certainly not always a bad thing. In fact, many people without GAD use it to help manage their worry. The problem arises when we use it frantically, out of fear—that is, to avoid what we fear will happen (e.g., going mad from worry). These fears need to be challenged and tested.

Another point to consider is how appropriate distraction is in different situations. Some people like to distract themselves by imagining pleasant things. While this may feel like an effective strategy, and even come naturally to some people, other people may really struggle to turn their mind to such things when they are distressed. Mentally removing yourself from the present moment can also impair your performance. Daydreaming about winning the lottery, while driving, may help you shift your attention away from worries, but it may also impair your driving ability! So, we would encourage you to turn you mind back to your present activity rather than distracting yourself with thoughts of things that are not currently happening.

Summary

In Section 5, we looked at beliefs about the costs and benefits of worrying, as well as how to practice letting go of worry. We used more thought challenging and experiments to tackle negative and positive beliefs about worry. Research suggests that these skills are very important in managing GAD. Keep up the good work. We wish you all the best!

Section 6: DEALING WITH BEHAVIORS THAT AFFECT WORRY

Recall that avoidance is the key behavior that keeps worry going. This section looks at how you can learn to reduce avoidance, one step at a time. Avoiding difficult things makes you feel more relaxed in the short term, but it is really unhelpful in the long term.

In Figure 6.5, you can see that when you confront a worrying situation, the anxiety will increase. By escaping or avoiding, the anxiety drops down. However, it just comes back again and again! Over time, the fear actually tends to grow. Avoidance perpetuates anxiety because it stops you finding out that your fears do not come true, or if they do, that you can cope.

In Section 2, we identified three main types of avoidance:

- Complete avoidance (e.g., avoiding places, people, activities)
- Safety behaviors—when people with GAD cannot completely avoid things, they often use subtle avoidance behaviors to prevent their fears from coming true (e.g., excessive checking, overplanning, being a perfectionist)
- Thought-control strategies—avoiding or controlling unpleasant thoughts (e.g., suppressing worry because you fear it will make you sick)

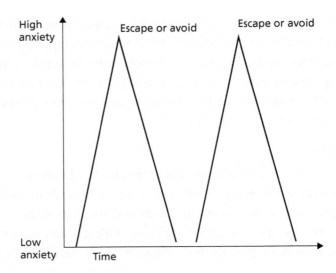

Figure 6.5 Avoidance maintains anxiety.

I've really become dependent on avoidance. It is stopping me doing things I want, and I know it is not a good way to deal with problems. I encourage my kids to face their fears and overcome them. I need to learn to do that, too.

In Figure 6.6, let us have a look at what will happen when you stop avoiding. Initially, your anxiety will increase, but if you let go of all forms of avoidance, your anxiety will gradually reduce. This reduction

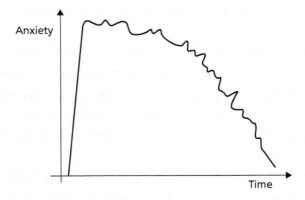

Figure 6.6 Anxiety reduces when you stop avoiding.

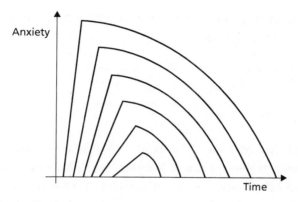

Figure 6.7 Desensitization over time

is often not a smooth experience—you will probably notice little ups and downs in the anxiety. However, bit by bit, the anxiety will reduce. It does this because you are becoming desensitized to the situation. You are finding out that your fears are not occurring and that you are coping. As you confront the same situation again and again, the anxiety gets less and less and does not last as long (see Figure 6.7).

It sounds so simple—too simple! Are you sure it works?

Yes, facing your fears is one of the best ways to overcome them. It is called "exposure." It is not an easy skill to master—it takes courage and persistence. You may need to confront your fears many times before the anxiety reduces.

But doesn't it make sense to avoid things that are dangerous?

Absolutely! If something is truly dangerous, we should avoid it. However, many of the things people with GAD avoid are not truly dangerous. In GAD, the excessive worry is like a false alarm going off when danger is not really present. If you are avoiding things that you used to do or that most people do on a regular basis, you are probably avoiding something that is not truly dangerous.

> I don't think I can do exposure . . . it sounds too hard!

Most people feel that way. That is why we take a very planned, gradual, and manageable approach. We start with situations that provoke a mild level of anxiety. You are in control of what you do and when you do it. This is NOT about throwing yourself in the deep end before you can swim properly! This is about building confidence and achieving your goals!

> How do I do exposure?

Graded exposure helps you face your fears one step at a time. We do this by constructing and completing "stepladders." There are five steps in this process:

Step 1. Write down your goal (e.g., to reduce avoidance and do things that you want to do).

Step 2. Make a list of activities and situations that are associated with your goal that trigger a range of anxiety from high to low. Be as specific as you can!

Step 3. Rate or rank the tasks from easy to hard (based on how anxious you expect to feel in the situation).

Step 4. Pick the easiest step and practice it *over and over again*, until you feel less anxious. Stay in the anxiety-producing situation as long as you can until your anxiety reduces substantially. Do not move up to the next step until you feel reasonably confident with this step.

Step 5. Move up to the next task. Repeat it over and over again until you feel less anxious and more confident. Treat each of your steps as an opportunity to find out if your worries come true and if you can cope.

Check out two of Liz's stepladders in Figure 6.8. (A blank form for you can be found at the end of this manual; see Form 6.9.)

Anxiety Level	**Goal: Doing everyday things to face my health worries**	**Goal: Letting go of control and my "need" for certainty**
VERY HIGH ANXIETY I can barely stand it	**VERY HIGH** ☐ Go to local hospital and walk around ☐ Watch movie about cancer/serious diseases/virus outbreaks ☐ Visit doctor once a month for a check-up or if I really am unwell. Don't go when I am panicking about cancer–wait a day so to see if I can cope on my own.	**VERY HIGH** ☐ Leaving my phone at home for the day ☐ Don't check emails before leaving work–leave on time ☐ Attend a dinner party where I don't know most people ☐ Let my husband take me away for a weekend–let him plan everything, don't ask any questions
HIGH ANXIETY My heart is racing	**HIGH** ☐ Don't seek reassurance from my husband that I am healthy ☐ Watch TV show about cancer/serious diseases ☐ Reduce hand washing to before eating and after using the toilet ☐ Go for a 10-minute run	**HIGH** ☐ Open mail every day, deal with it straight away (or write in my diary as appropriate) ☐ Don't ask assistant to remind me to do things–look in diary once a day ☐ Have friends come over for lunch. Ask them to bring something and arrive 'whenever'
MEDIUM Unpleasant; I really don't want to be here	**MEDIUM** ☐ Stop checking internet about possible diagnosis for symptoms I have ☐ Eat in a food court ☐ Go to http://www.healthtalk.org/ and hear people stories of cancer/serious disease	**MEDIUM** ☐ Go shopping without a list ☐ Delegate minor tasks to Dave ☐ Go to a new restaurant and order something new from a menu
LOW- MILD ANXIETY I'm aware of my tension, but I can handle this	**LOW** ☐ Stop checking my body every day for lumps/spots (do once a month) ☐ Watch TV ads about smoking, drinking, health (don't change the channel) ☐ Read a fact sheets on cancer from the Cancer Society	**LOW** ☐ Let kids decide what we will do one weekend ☐ Limit meeting preparation to 30 minutes ☐ After Friday review meetings, use the problem-solving technique to make decisions rather than procrastinating ☐ Saying hello to a shop assistant
VERY LOW- –A bit of tension; I'm fine, this just feels a bit odd	**VERY LOW** ☐ Go for 5-minute fast walk–feel a bit faint and have palpitations ☐ Stop avoiding Charlie-his mum had cancer ☐ Eat foods that I would normally avoid (e.g., sushi)	**VERY LOW** ☐ Stop asking my assistant "Are we on top of everything?" ☐ Don't check my phone/email for 1hour ☐ Limit meeting preparation to 1 hour

Figure 6.8 Liz's stepladders.

Tips!

Watch out for safety behaviors and thought-control strategies

Safety behaviors and thought-control strategies (e.g., suppressing worry, being self-critical, reassuring yourself) are unhelpful during exposure. They are more forms of avoidance and can reduce the effectiveness of your exposure. Try to stay focused on the present during exposure so that you can test if your fears come true. If you struggle to do exposure without safety behaviors, drop them off as soon as possible, or break the step down into more manageable tasks so that you do not rely on safety behaviors.

What do I base my stepladder on?

◆ Try looking back at Section 2 where you identified your typical avoidance behaviors.

◆ Think about what you want to do, but are held back by the worry and anxiety.

◆ Consider these common ones:

- Improving assertiveness—saying no, giving opinions, stating your decisions, limiting excessive apologizing, stop seeking reassurance
- Being more flexible—reducing perfectionism and excessive responsibility taking, learning to be comfortable making mistakes and not having a plan B, delegating tasks, reducing excessive checking, allowing others to do things for themselves
- Social situations—conversations, entertaining, being the centre of attention, performing, making new friends/reconnecting with old friends
- Targeting specific fears—heights, dogs, driving, new places.

What if my anxiety does not reduce with repeated exposure?

That is okay. There are lots of reasons why this may be happening. You may not have stayed in the situation long enough for the anxiety to reduce or for you to find out if your worries were true. The task may be too hard—you will need to break the step down into two or three easier steps. Then repeat the easier steps on several occasions. On the other hand, you may have been using safety behaviors. These often prevent you from coping on your own and keep the anxiety going over time. Lastly, was your attention focused on the moment? Or were you "catastrophizing" during the situation? Thinking the worst (rather than focusing on what is really happening) will keep you feeling anxious.

It all seems too hard. Help!

Do not think about the steps at the top of your ladder. Focus on the first step. If that seems too big, it is not the first step! Try breaking it down even further. The important thing is to get started—so let go of criticizing yourself, dismissing your efforts, or wanting to do things "perfectly." You might like to get some help from a friend or clinician.

How often do you do exposure?

To begin with, you may need to set aside specific times during your week to practice a step—we suggest you aim for at least three times in a week. This repetition, within a brief space of time, will give you a good chance to learn something new. However, as you build your confidence, we hope you will be doing exposure every day! We hope you will develop an attitude where you want to approach and solve your difficulties, rather than avoid them.

> Exposure stepladders are not easy—but they do work! I didn't think I could do them. I had to keep reminding myself that getting better was not a race. I have been anxious most of my life, so my worries were not going to vanish overnight.
>
> I have been working on my stepladders for about three months now. I have come to realize that I can deal with difficult situations. I used to think that coping meant feeling confident all the time and not feeling stressed at all—like in fairy tales, living happily ever after. I don't think that anymore. For me, coping is about doing difficult things when you need to and you want to—even if that means feeling upset and frightened.
>
> I still have a long way to go in facing my fears, but I'll get there . . . and so can you!

Summary

In Section 6, we saw that facing your fears through exposure tasks is a good way to address the behavioral symptoms of GAD. Changing your behavior takes time and effort, but it will build your confidence and help you master your worry. Aim to build these skills gradually over the next few weeks. All the best!

Section 7: ADVANCED SKILLS FOR FACING FEARS

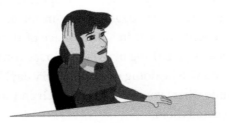

I can't work out how to build a stepladder for some of my worries, like dying of a brain tumor, my son getting kidnapped, or my husband dying in a car crash. I figured out ways to reduce some of my safety behaviors for these worries—like reducing my reassurance seeking—but how do you exposure yourself to dying of a brain tumor? It sounds ridiculous!

Great question Liz! We use "imaginal exposure" to tackle worries about catastrophic events or hypothetical problems (i.e., problems that are not occurring currently or in the foreseeable future). Imaginal exposure involves gradually imagining the "worst case scenario" and exposing yourself to the mental images, thoughts, emotions, and physical sensations associated with the worry. Like other steps on your stepladder, when you repeatedly exposure yourself to these things, you become desensitized to the fear, and your sense of being able to cope grows.

Imagining the worst case scenario . . . I think I do that already when I worry. Why haven't I desensitized myself to these fears yet?

Research has shown that imaginal exposure is actually quite different from worrying. During imaginal exposure, you are actively scheduling in time to directly face your fears, rather than just worrying about things at random times. It encourages you to follow your worries through to their conclusion rather than "jumping out" of them with safety behaviors (e.g., reassuring yourself, distracting yourself, suppressing your thoughts) when they get too confronting. This actually allows you to emotionally process distressing images and feelings and, as a result, you can "desensitize" or get used to them.

> But these situations are my worst nightmares. I'd rather not think about them at all!

That is completely understandable but has trying not to think about these things helped you cope with them?

> Not really. I guess that's just more avoidance. The more I try to not think about these things, the more they are in my mind.

That is right. However, the good news is that the more exposure you do to these "worst case scenarios," the less they will bother you and the more you will be able to cope with the thought of them.

> Well that sounds good. I'm still not sure, but I'll give it a try. How do I do imaginal exposure?

There is a six-step process you can follow:

Step 1. Select a worry to work on. It needs to be about a possible future catastrophe or disaster, rather than a specific problem that you are experiencing at the moment. For example, a future disaster could involve becoming destitute and friendless, whereas a current problem may be having unsupportive friends at the moment. If you have a range of worries, pick the easiest one to face first.

Step 2. Identify the most feared outcome or "worst case scenario." This is often not pleasant to do, but it is an essential step. Ask yourself "What am I most worried will happen? What is the absolute worst thing that could happen?" Write it down.

Step 3. Imaginal exposure. This can be done in a couple of ways and can be graded—that is, start with something easier at first, then progress to a more difficult task when you are ready.

One way to do imaginal exposure is to close your eyes and create an image or picture in your mind of the worst possible outcome. See it in your mind's eye as vividly as possible—picture what is happening in detail, with all the sounds, smells, tastes, and feelings that you can evoke. Allow any unpleasant feelings to come and go. Do not distract yourself in any way. If your mind starts to wonder, look at what you wrote down (Step 2) and refocus back on the image. Continue doing this for 25 minutes (set an alarm to go off so you do not distract yourself by watching the time).

Table 6.14 Liz's imaginal exposure

Steps	Liz's exposure
Step 1. Select a worry.	Having a headache (or stomach ache) and getting really sick
Step 2. Identify the worst case scenario.	Dying of cancer
Step 3. Hold the image in your mind for 25 minutes as vividly as possible. Do not distract yourself in any way.	The image I held in my mind: "I am lying in a hospital bed with my family around me. My kids are crying. My husband is weeping and holding my hand. He is saying 'we'll all be OK' but I know I am dying. I can't move, the pain is everywhere— it makes it hard to breathe. The nurses and doctors scurry around me, shaking their heads and sighing. They put needles in my arms. The machines beep and the smell of disinfectant makes me feel sick. I feel the life slip away from me. Everything is black."
Step 4. Beside the worst case outcome, what else could happen?	◆ I get a headache/stomach ache and it passes in time. ◆ I get a headache/stomach ache and I take paracetamol and it goes away. ◆ I get sick but my GP prescribes medication and I get better. ◆ I get sick and get admitted to hospital but eventually get better. ◆ I get cancer; it is treated; I get better and continue living.
Step 5. Reflect on your experiences.	I felt very anxious and sad imagining the worst outcome, but the longer I did it, the easier it got. I worried that thinking about it would make it happen, and I was very tempted to distract or reassure myself. The alternative outcomes seem much more likely to me.
Step 6. Repeat the exposure	I repeated this exposure every day for a week. By the last day, my anxiety had reduced from very high to moderate. I will keep going for another week.

Another way to do imaginal exposure is to write a "worry story" about how the worst possible outcome occurs. Write the story as though it is happening now and from your perspective (e.g., "I feel …," "I see …"). Describe in vivid detail what happens and how you feel. As you write, allow images and emotions to surface. Do nothing either to distract yourself or to get rid of distressing thoughts and feelings. Try to write a few paragraphs and do not end your story before the catastrophic outcome is reached.

Step 4. Open your eyes and/or focus your attention back to the here and now. Now, write down all the other outcomes that could occur besides the worst possible outcome. That is, generate a variety of alternative events that could come to pass that do not involve the worst case scenario. List everything you could do to cope and/or marshal support to prevent the worst outcome occurring.

Step 5. Take a moment to reflect on what the imaginal exposure was like for you. How did you feel? Did your feelings change across the exercise? How so? How likely do you feel the worst case scenario is compared to the alternative outcomes?

Step 6. Repeat the imaginal exposure until your anxiety reduces. Keep a record of your experiences as you repeat the exposure.

Table 6.14 shows one of Liz's imaginal exposure records. (A blank record for you can be found at the end of this manual; see Form 6.10.)

> Instead of imagining a scene in my head, sometimes I wrote a "worry story" about my worst fears coming true. Here is my story about my son, Adam.

Liz's worry story: My son being kidnapped

"I am sitting at home. The kids are a bit late coming home from school. There is a knock at the door—two policemen are there with my daughter, Lilly. She is crying and fear suddenly grips my heart. The police tell me that my children were attacked. Lilly managed to escape, but Adam was taken by a man in a dark car. Lilly is sobbing and clinging to me for dear life. She is so frightened. I start to panic; I don't know what to do. Where is Adam? He must be terrified. What is happening to him? I can't cope with the doubt. I am to blame. I should have been more careful.

I feel there is no hope. Adam is gone forever; I have lost my son. Jim will be
   devastated—his only son is gone. Lilly will be scarred for life. I hate
   the man who took Adam. I want him dead. I feel like I will pass out.
The weeks and months go by, but still the police haven't found Adam.
   I am becoming more and more depressed. Lilly and Jim can't
   cope. The grief overwhelms us all. We don't feel like a family any-
   more. The doubt and uncertainty about where Adam is tears me
   apart. I feel so guilty, sad, and angry.
Finally, we get the news. Adam's body has been found. My poor sweet
   boy; I wish it had happened to me. I feel totally numb and empty.
   My heart breaks completely; I know I will never be happy again."

After writing the story several times, my anxiety changed (see Table 6.15).

Table 6.15 Repeating imaginal exposure

First and second time writing the story	Fifth and sixth time writing the story	Ninth and tenth time writing the story
◆ Strong feelings of guilt, sadness, and anxiety ◆ Had to work hard to not try and reassure myself that the event would not happen ◆ Had to work hard to write the story to the end (worry that if I write it, it will come true) Anxiety: 100/100	◆ Feelings of guilt, sadness, and anxiety, but not as strong as before ◆ Helped identify that some of my daily worries stem from this worst case scenario ◆ Emotions passed sooner than first two attempts and I feel that this story is really not likely to come true; it is far more likely that Adam will be safe walking home from school with Lilly and his friends Anxiety: 60/100	◆ Able to write the story and acknowledge that the events in the story are horrible and I would not want it to happen ◆ But, was able to sit with the anxiety and not be overwhelmed by emotions or other thoughts ◆ I am not happy at the end of my story, but I am starting to see that if it were to happen, that I could possibly cope somehow Anxiety: 30/100

Summary

Section 7 has shown you how to face your worries through imaginal
exposure. This type of exposure is particularly useful for worries about
situations that are not happening at the present time and involve threatening but unlikely events. Imaginal exposure is confronting but, as with
any form of exposure, the more you practice it, the easier it becomes.
For some people with GAD, it is the main form of exposure they use.

We would encourage you to try imaginal exposure over the next few
weeks. Good luck and we will see you again soon!

Section 8: PUTTING IT ALL TOGETHER AND STAYING WELL IN THE LONGER TERM

Congratulations, you have almost finished the GAD Program! In this final section of the program, we look at some ways to maintain the gains you have made and how to progress further.

First, let us review the key skills you have seen during this program. Each skill corresponds to the symptom types that make up GAD (and keep it going). Remember the diagram of thoughts, physical sensations, or behaviors (see Figure 6.9)?

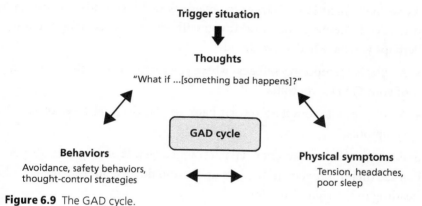

Figure 6.9 The GAD cycle.

Skills toolbox

Strategies to manage physical symptoms:

- Medication
- Controlled breathing
- Progressive muscle relaxation
- Exercise

Strategies to manage the thought symptoms:

- Recognizing unhelpful thinking patterns
- Thought-challenging records
- Worry experiments

- Structured problem solving
- Recognizing and challenging negative and positive beliefs about worry
- Letting go of worries and keeping active

Strategies to manage the behavioral symptoms:

- Facing your fears via exposure stepladders
- Imaginal exposure and worry stories
- Dropping safety behaviors

Lapses and relapses explained

As we have mentioned earlier, recovery is not a smooth process. As you learn to manage your worry, you will have setbacks along the way. Perhaps you have had a few already.

- A *lapse* is a temporary setback, where you experience a return of some of your GAD symptoms.
- A *relapse* is a complete return back to the original level of GAD symptoms.

Setbacks and lapses are a normal part of recovery. From Figure 6.10, you can see that improvement has lots of ups and downs, but the line is still heading in the right direction.

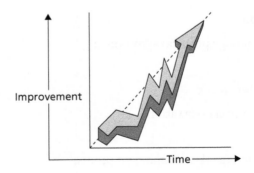

Figure 6.10 Setbacks are normal.

So is there any way to know when you will have a lapse?

Lapses tend to occur at certain times, which include the following:

♦ When people stop practicing and using their new skills.

♦ When people experience stressful things in their life. These can include stressful events like starting a new job, moving house, beginning a new relationship or ending an old relationship, the death of a friend or family member, financial problems, and so on.

♦ When people experience periods of change in their lives or when daily routines are altered, such as retirement, having a child, or taking holidays.

♦ When we are unwell, tired, or overwhelmed. At these times, managing worry is harder and you may find yourself at greater risk of a lapse.

So what do you do when you have a lapse?

Here is a list of things we encourage you to do when you have a setback:

♦ Avoid catastrophizing about the setback and being self-critical (e.g., "I'm back to square one. I'm hopeless. I can't do anything right. I'll be like this forever!"). Remind yourself that lapses are normal; they are to be expected and they do not mean that you have failed.

♦ Identify why the lapse may have occurred (e.g., Did you stop practicing your skills? Did life suddenly become more stressful than usual? Did you try to confront a situation that was too high on your exposure stepladder?)

♦ Remember that your symptoms did not arrive overnight, so they will not go away overnight. You may have been a worrier for many, many years.

♦ Remember the progress that you have made, despite the setback, and give yourself a pat on the back for it.

♦ Do not be perfectionistic about the lapse—show the same compassion to yourself that you would show to a close friend or loved one.

♦ Get some extra help from family and friends, or doctors and other clinicians.

♦ Remind yourself that you still have important CBT skills. Put your relapse prevention plan into action.

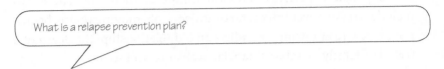

What is a relapse prevention plan?

This is a practical guide to reducing your risk of relapse and to deal with setbacks. There are three straightforward steps to follow to put your plan together.

Step 1. Identify your early warning signs

Recognizing early warning signs is very important. If you can identify the first signs that the worry is getting out of hand, you can deal with it quickly.

Early warning signs are subtle symptoms of GAD that indicate the problem is returning. They are often things like spending more time worrying, feeling more tense than normal, or starting to avoid things again. Take some time to record what your early warning signs are likely to be (see Table 6.16).

Table 6.16 Early warning signs of relapse

Symptoms	My early warning signs
Thoughts/ worries	
Physical signs	
Behaviors	

Step 2. Get proactive!

As soon as you notice some early warning signs, revise your CBT skills. Look back over your skills toolkit and start to challenge worries, practice relaxation skills, and face your fears again. You will need to make time to use your skills. Do not give up! If they have helped before, they will help again.

If you think it would be beneficial, get some extra help from family, friends, your doctor, or psychologist.

> My doctor is helpful, but I don't always need to see her—most times talking to a friend helps me relax and put things into perspective.

Step 3. Develop and work towards goals

These are goals for staying well and progressing further towards your recovery. Liz's goals for keeping on track and getting even better are:

- Schedule time every month to review my GAD workbook
- Make a new stepladder when I finish an old one
- Take time off regularly for relaxation and exercise
- Practice realistic thinking regularly
- Ask my husband and best friend to tell me when I am starting to worry too much again

Write down your ideas and plans here:

1.

2.

3.

4.

5.

6.

Where can I get more information about managing anxiety?

If you would like to read more about managing worry with CBT, we would suggest the following books:

- *Mastery of your anxiety worry* by Michelle Craske and David Barlow
- *Take control of your worry* by Lisa Lampe
- *The anti-anxiety workbook: proven strategies to overcome worry, phobias, panic, and obsessions* by Martin Anthony and Peter Norton
- *It's not all in your head: how worrying about your health could be making you sick—and what you can do about it* by Gordon Asmundson and Steven Taylor
- *Overcoming perfectionism* by Roz Shafran, Sarah Egan, and Tracey Wade
- *Mind over mood* by Dennis Greenberger and Christine Padesky
- *Beating the blues* by Susan Tanner and Jillian Ball

You may also find the following websites helpful:

- Clinical Research Unit for Anxiety and Depression: http://www.crufad.com/
- Centre for Clinical Interventions: http://www.cci.health.wa.gov.au/
- Cognitive Behaviour Therapy Self-Help Resources: http://www.getselfhelp.co.uk/

In conclusion ...

We hope you have found this program helpful. Learning to manage your worry can be a very difficult and challenging process, but it can also be rewarding and liberating.

Congratulations again for all your hard work! We wish you all the best for your future!

Record forms for patients

Form 6.3 Worry log

Date and situation	Feelings and physical symptoms What did I feel and what happened in my body?	Thoughts What went through my mind?	Behaviors What did I do?

Progressive muscle relaxation exercises

Find a quiet place where you will not be interrupted. Sit comfortably in a chair with back and arm support, or lie on the floor if this is more comfortable for you. Allow about 15 minutes for these exercises. Do not worry if your mind wanders during the exercises—this is normal. Just try to let go of the thought that has distracted you and bring your attention gently back to the exercises that you are doing.

Beginning exercises

- Close your eyes, if you are comfortable doing so.
- Become aware of your breathing. Notice when you breathe in and out. Breathe through your nose slowly and gently. Aim to breathe with your diaphragm (rather than your chest).
- Notice the feeling of the breath as it passes through your nose and into your body. Notice the rise and fall of your stomach or chest as you gently breathe in and out.
- On each out breath, encourage yourself to relax. Continue this for a few minutes.

Progressive muscle relaxation

There are three steps to do as you work your way around your body. First, bring awareness to the part of the body. Second, apply tension. Tense to the point that it is noticeable; the exercises should not be uncomfortable or painful. Third, release tension and relax. After each muscle group, take a minute to relax and breathe. Follow this order:

Feet and toes	1. Become aware: what do they feel like? Warm, cool, heavy, tingling?
	2. Tense (5 seconds): curl your toes under your feet.
	3. Release (10 seconds): relax the tension; with each out breath, relax more and more. Gently tell yourself to relax.
Lower legs and thighs	1. Become aware: what do they feel like? Is there tension?
	2. Tense (5 seconds): push your heels into the floor.
	3. Release (10 seconds): again, breathe slowly and smoothly, encouraging yourself to relax each time you breathe out.

Bottom and back	1. Become aware: notice any tension. 2. Tense (5 seconds): gently tighten the muscles in your bottom and push your back into the chair or floor. 3. Release (10 seconds): slowly relax these muscles; relax more with each breath. Let them go loose and floppy.
Shoulders and neck	1. Become aware: are you holding tension there? 2. Tense (5 seconds): lift up your shoulders towards your ears and pull your chin closer into your chest. 3. Release (10 seconds): drop your shoulders and lengthen your neck. With each out breath, drop and loosen your shoulders more and more.
Fingers, hands, and arms	1. Become aware: what do they feel like? Warm, cool, heavy, tingling? 2. Tense (5 seconds): making fists with your hands and lifting your arms out in front of you. 3. Release (10 seconds): allow your hands to relax and your arms to rest gently on your lap or on the floor. Breathe out any tension.
Face and head	1. Become aware: notice the sensations in your lips, cheeks, eyelids, nose, forehead, and scalp. 2. Tense (5 seconds): gently clench your jaw, screw up your nose, purse your lips, close your eyes more tightly, and furrow your brow. 3. Release (10 seconds): relax all these muscles. Notice the difference between the tense and relaxed feelings.

Finishing exercises

- Bring your awareness back to your breath. Ensure your breathing is slow, smooth, and soft. With each out breath, we again encourage you to relax and let go of any tension.

- Scan your body for any sources of tension. Start with your feet, work up through your legs and back, through to your shoulders, arms, neck, face, and head. Release any tension or tightness you find.

- Keep breathing slowly and enjoy the feeling of relaxation.

- When you are ready, slowly wiggle your fingers and toes. Open your eyes and bring your attention to where you are.

Form 6.4 Monitoring relaxation exercises

Date and time	Tension before (0–100)	Tension after (0–100)	Reflections What was that like? What parts of your body are easiest or hardest to relax? What happened in your mind or to your worry during relaxation?

Form 6.5 Thought-challenging record

Identify the situation and recognize your thoughts	Test whether your thoughts are realistic (use the list of questions in Section 4)	Shift thoughts to be more realistic and helpful
Situation: Thoughts:		What experiment could you conduct to test this worry out?
	Unhelpful thinking patterns:	What happened?

Form 6.6 Structured problem-solving worksheet

Step 1. What is the problem/goal? Carefully think about what the problem is—the more narrowly you can define it, the better.	
Step 2. List all possible solutions. Put down all ideas, even bad ones!	
Step 3. Evaluate each possible solution. *Quickly* go down the list of solutions and consider the advantages and disadvantages of each. **Choose a solution.** Pick the best solution; try to pick one that you can start to work on straight away.	
Step 4. Plan how to carry out the solution. Plan out, step by step, what you will do.	
Step 5. Review progress. Focus on the things you have achieved and be pleased with any progress you have made. Consider what needs to be done next.	

Form 6.7 Thought record for negative beliefs about worry

Identify the negative belief about your worry	Test whether your belief is realistic (use the list of questions in Section 5)	Change the belief to be more realistic and helpful
Belief: **Clarify what this belief means to you.** If this belief was true, and you worried a lot, what do you fear would happen?		**What experiment could you conduct to test this belief?** **What happened?**

Form 6.8 Thought record for positive beliefs about worry

Identify the positive belief about worry	Test whether your belief is realistic (use the list of questions in Section 5)	Change the belief to be more realistic and helpful
Belief: **Clarify what this belief means to you.** If this belief was true, and you worried a lot, what would happen?		**What experiment could you conduct to test this belief?** **What happened?**

Form 6.9 Exposure stepladders

Anxiety Level	Goal:	Goal:
VERY HIGH ANXIETY I can barely stand it	VERY HIGH	VERY HIGH
HIGH ANXIETY My hear is racing	HIGH	HIGH
MEDIUM Unpleasant I really don't want to be here	MEDIUM	MEDIUM
LOW Mild anxiety: I'm aware of my tension, but I can handle this	LOW	LOW
VERY LOW A bit of tension I'm fine, this just feels a bit odd	VERY LOW	VERY LOW

Form 6.10 Imaginal exposure log

Steps	
Step 1. Select a worry.	
Step 2. Identify the worst case scenario.	
Step 3. Hold the image in your mind for 25 minutes as vividly as possible. Do not distract yourself in any way.	
Step 4. Beside the worst case outcome, what else could happen?	
Step 5. Reflect on your experiences.	
Step 6. Repeat the exposure.	

Finding answers to common questions

Table 6.17 Finding answers to common questions

Common questions	Read
Understanding GAD and treatment	Sections 1 & 2
I have been told I may have GAD. What is it?	
Why can I not stop worrying? What causes GAD and what keeps it going?	
What is CBT?	
Should I take medication? I do not want to get addicted.	
I am not sure how my worry impacts on my everyday life.	
Dealing with physical symptoms	Section 3
I need help relaxing.	
How do I calm down by breathing more slowly?	
I have heard exercise helps anxiety. Got any tips?	
Shifting what you think	Sections 4 & 5
I tend to think the worst all the time. How can I be less pessimistic?	
I just keep thinking that I cannot cope!	
People tell me to not worry so much, but worry can be helpful—can it not?	
My worries seem a bit silly, but I just cannot let them go. Got any tips?	
I cannot stand not being in control and not knowing what is going to happen.	
I worry a lot about my worrying. Is worry really damaging?	
I think I am going crazy! Am I?	
I feel better, but what if my worry comes back?	
I can challenge my negative thinking, but my new thoughts are not very convincing!	
Changing what you do	Sections 6 & 7
Worry really stops me doing what I want to do.	
The more I push my worries away, the more they come back!	
I put off dealing with my problems and tasks.	
I am a bit of a perfectionist and a control freak. How can I change some of the things I do?	
I check and seek reassurance too much.	
I worry about dreadful things. They are not likely to happen, but how can I cope with these fears?	

References

Akiskal, H. S. (1998). Toward a definition of generalized anxiety disorder as an anxious temperament type. *Acta Psychiatrica Scandinavica, 393*, 66–73.

Alegria, M., Takeuchi, D., Canino, G., Duan, N., Shrout, P., Meng, X. -L., ... Gong, F. (2004). Considering context, place and culture: the National Latino and Asian American Study. *International Journal of Methods in Psychiatric Research, 13*, 208–220.

American Psychiatric Association. (2013). *Diagnostic and statistical manual for mental disorders* (5th ed.). Washington, DC: American Psychiatric Association.

Andersson, G., Paxling, B., Roch-Norlund, P., Ostman, G., Norgren, A., Almlov, J., ... Silverberg, F. (2012). Internet-based psychodynamic versus cognitive behavioural guided self-help for generalized anxiety disorder: a randomized controlled trial. *Psychotherapy and Psychosomatics, 81*, 344–355.

Andreescu, C., Gross, J. J., Lenze, E., Edelman, K. D., Snyder, S., Tanase, C., & Aizenstein, H. (2011). Altered cerebral blood flow patterns associated with pathologic worry in the elderly. *Depression and Anxiety, 28*, 202–209.

Andrews, G. (1996). Comorbidity and the general neurotic syndrome. *British Journal of Psychiatry, 168*(Suppl. 30), S76–S84.

Andrews, G., Creamer, M., Crino, R., Hunt, C., Lampe, L., & Page, A. (2003). *The treatment of anxiety disorders: clinician guides and patient manuals*. Cambridge, UK: Cambridge University Press.

Andrews, G., Cuijpers, P., Craske, M., McEvoy, P., & Titov, N. (2010b). Computer therapy for the anxiety and depressive disorders is effective, acceptable and practical health care: a meta-analysis. *PLoS One, 5*(10), e13196.

Andrews, G., Dean, K., Genderson, M., Hunt, C., Mitchell, P., Sachdev, P. S., & Trollor, J. N. (2013). *Management of mental disorders* (5th ed.). Sydney: Amazon. com.

Andrews, G., Goldberg, D. P., Krueger, R. F., Carpenter, W. T., Hyman, S. E., Sachdev, P. S., & Pine, D. S. (2009a). Exploring the feasibility of a meta-structure for DSM-V and ICD-11: could it improve utility and validity? *Psychological Medicine, 39*, 1993–2000.

Andrews, G., Hobbs, M. J., Borkovec, T. D., Beesdo, K., Craske, M. G., Heimberg, R. G., ... Stanley, M. A. (2010a). Generalized worry disorder: a review of DSM-IV generalized anxiety disorder and options for DSM-V. *Depression and Anxiety, 27*, 134–147.

Andrews, G., Pine, D. S., Hobbs, M. J., Anderson, T. M., & Sunderland, M. (2009b). Neurodevelopmental disorders: Cluster 2 of the proposed meta-structure for DSM-V. *Psychological Medicine, 39*, 2013–2023.

Angst, J., Gamma, A., Baldwin, D. S., Ajdacic-Gross, V., & Rössler, W. (2009). The generalized anxiety spectrum: prevalence, onset, course and outcome. *European Archives of Psychiatry and Clinical Neuroscience, 259,* 37–45.

Angst, J., Gamma, A., Bienvenu, O. J., Eaton, W. W., Adjacic, V., Eich, D., & Rössler, W. (2006). Varying temporal criteria for generalized anxiety disorder: prevalence and clinical characteristics in a young age cohort. *Psychological Medicine, 36,* 1283–1292.

Arntz, A. (2003). Cognitive therapy versus applied relaxation as treatment of generalized anxiety disorder. *Behaviour Research and Therapy, 41,* 633–646.

Asmundson, G. J. G., Fetzner, M. G., DeBoer, L. B., Powers, M. B., Otto, M. W., & Smits, J. A. J. (2013). Let's get physical: a contemporary review of the anxiolytic effects of exercise for anxiety and its disorders. *Depression and Anxiety, 30,* 362–373.

Aviram, A. & Westra, H. A. (2011). The impact of motivational interviewing on resistance in cognitive behavioural therapy for generalized anxiety disorder. *Psychotherapy Research, 21*(6), 698–708.

Baldwin, D. S., Woods, R., Lawson, R., & Taylor, D. (2011). Efficacy of drug treatments for generalized anxiety disorder: systematic review and meta-analysis. *British Medical Journal, 342,* 637–648.

Baldwin, D. S., Waldman, S., & Allgulander, C. (2011). Evidence-based pharmacological treatment of generalized anxiety disorder. *International Journal of Neuropsychopharmacology, 14,* 697–710.

Ballenger, J. C., Davidson, J. R. T., Lecrubier, Y., Nutt, D. J., Borkovec, T. D., Rickels, K., … Wittchen, H. -U. (2001). Consensus statement on generalized anxiety disorder from the International Consensus Group on Depression and Anxiety. *Journal of Clinical Psychiatry, 62*(Suppl. 11), S53–S58.

Barlow, D. H. (1985). The dimensions of anxiety disorders. In A. H. Tuma & J. D. Maser (Eds.), *Anxiety and the anxiety disorders* (pp. 479–500). Hillsdale, NJ: Lawrence Erlbaum Associates.

Barlow, D. H., Blanchard, E. B., Vermilyea, B. B., Vermilyea, J. A., & Di Nardo, P. A. (1986a). Generalized anxiety and generalized anxiety disorder: description and reconceptualization. *American Journal of Psychiatry, 143,* 40–44.

Barlow, D. H., Di Nardo, P. A., Vermilyea, B. B., & Blanchard, E. B. (1986b). Co-morbidity and depression among the anxiety disorders: issues in diagnosis and classification. *Journal of Nervous Mental Disease, 174,* 63–72.

Barlow, D. H., Farchione, T. J., Fairholme, C. P., Ellard, K. K., Boisseau, C. L, Allen, L. B., & Ehrenreich May, J. T. (2011). *Unified protocol for transdiagnostic treatment of emotional disorders: therapist guide (treatments that work).* New York: Oxford University Press.

Beesdo-Baum, K., Jenjahn, E., Hofler, M., Lueken, U., Becker, E. S., & Hoyer, J. (2012). Avoidance, safety behaviour, and reassurance seeking in generalized anxiety disorder. *Depression and Anxiety, 29,* 948–957.

Beesdo-Baum, K., Winkel, S., Pine, D. S., Hoyer, J., Höfler, M., Lieb, R., & Wittchen, H. -U. (2011). The diagnostic threshold of generalized anxiety disorder in the community: a developmental perspective. *Journal of Psychiatric Research*, *45*, 962–972.

Behar, E. & Borkovec, T. D. (2005). The nature and treatment of generalized anxiety disorder. In B. O. Rothbaum (Ed.), *The nature and treatment of pathological anxiety: essays in honor of Edna B. Foa* (pp. 181–196). New York: Guilford.

Behar, E., Di Marco, I. D., Hekler, E. B., Mohlman, J., & Staples, A. M. (2009). Current theoretical models of generalized anxiety disorder (GAD): conceptual review and treatment implications. *Journal of Anxiety Disorders, 23,* 1011–1023.

Berle, D., Starcevic, V., Moses, K., Hannan, A., Milicevic, D., & Sammut, P. (2011). Preliminary validation of an ultra-brief version of the Penn State Worry Questionnaire. *Clinical Psychology and Psychotherapy, 18,* 339–346.

Berstein, D. A. & Borkovec, T. D. (1973). *Progressive muscle training: a manual for the helping professions*. Champaign, IL: Research Press.

Bienvenu, O. J., Nestadt, G., & Eaton, W. W. (1998). Characterizing generalized anxiety: temporal and symptomatic thresholds. *Journal of Nervous Mental Disorders, 186,* 51–56.

Bond, F. W., Hayes, S. C., Baer, R. A., Carpenter, K. M., Guenole, N., Orcutt, H. K., … Zette, R. D. (2011). Preliminary psychometric properties of the Acceptance and Action Questionnaire-II: a revised measure of psychological inflexibility and experiential avoidance. *Behaviour Therapy, 42,* 676–688.

Borkovec, T. D., Abel, J. A., & Newman, H. (1995). Effects of psychotherapy on comorbid conditions in generalized anxiety disorder. *Journal of Consulting and Clinical Psychology, 63,* 479–483.

Borkovec, T. D., Alcaine, O. M., & Behar, E. (2004). Avoidance theory of worry and generalized anxiety disorder. In R. G. Heimberg, C. L. Turk, & D. Mennin (Eds.), *Generalized anxiety disorder: advances in research and practice*. New York, NY: Guilford Press.

Borkovec, T. D. & Costello, E. J. (1993). Efficacy of applied relaxation and cognitive behavioural therapy in the treatment of generalized anxiety disorder. *Journal of Consulting and Clinical Psychology, 61,* 611–619.

Borkovec, T. D. & Hu, S. (1990). The effect of worry on cardiovascular response to phobic imagery. *Behaviour Research and Therapy, 28,* 69–73.

Borkovec, T. D. & Inz, J. (1990). The nature of worry in generalized anxiety disorder: a predominance of thought activity. *Behaviour Research and Therapy, 28,* 153–158.

Borkovec, T. D., Newman, M. G., Pincus, A. L., & Lytle, R. (2002). A component analysis of cognitive-behavioural therapy for generalized anxiety disorder and the role of interpersonal problems. *Journal of Consulting and Clinical Psychology, 70,* 288–298.

Borkovec, T. D. & Roemer, L. (1995). Perceived functions of worry among generalized anxiety disorder subjects: distraction from more emotionally distressing topics? *Journal of Behaviour Therapy and Experimental Psychiatry, 26*(1), 25–30.

Boschen, M. J. (2011). A meta-analysis of the efficacy of pregabalin in the treatment of generalized anxiety disorder. *Canadian Journal of Psychiatry, 56*, 558–566.

Boswell, J. F., Thompson-Hollands, J., Farchione, T. J., & Barlow, D. H. (2013). Intolerance of uncertainty: a common factor in the treatment of emotional disorders. *Journal of Clinical Psychology, 69*, 630–645.

Brawman-Mintzer, O., Lydiard, R. B., Emmanuel, N., Payeur, R., Johnson, M., Roberts, J., … Ballenger, J. C. (1993). Psychiatric comorbidity in patients with generalized anxiety disorder. *American Journal of Psychiatry, 150*, 1216–1218.

Brosschot, J. F., Gerin, W., & Thayer, J. F. (2006). The perseverative cognition hypothesis: a review of worry, prolonged stress-related physiological activation, and health. *Journal of Psychosomatic Research, 60*(2), 113–124.

Brown, T. A., Antony, M. M., & Barlow, D. H. (1992). Psychometric properties of the Penn State Worry Questionnaire in a clinical anxiety disorder sample. *Behaviour Research and Therapy, 30*, 33–37.

Brown, T. A. & Barlow, D. H. (1992). Comorbidity among anxiety disorders: implications for treatment and DSM-IV. *Journal of Consulting and Clinical Psychology, 60*, 835–844.

Brown, T. A., Barlow, D. H., & Liebowitz, M. R. (1994). The empirical basis of generalized anxiety disorder. *American Journal of Psychiatry 151*, 1272–1280.

Brown, T. A., Campbell, L. A., Lehman, C. L., Grisham, J. R., & Mancill, R. B. (2001a). Current and lifetime comorbidity of the DSM-IV anxiety and mood disorders in a large clinical sample. *Journal of Abnormal Psychology, 110*, 49–58.

Brown, T. A., Chorpita, B. F., & Barlow, D. H. (1998). Structural relationships among dimensions of the DSM-IV anxiety and mood disorders and dimensions of negative affect, positive affect, and autonomic arousal. *Journal of Abnormal Psychology, 107*, 179–192.

Brown, T. A., Di Nardo, P. A., & Barlow, D. H. (1994). *Anxiety disorders interview schedule for DSM-IV*. New York, NY: Oxford University Press.

Brown, T. A., Di Nardo, P. A., Lehman, C. L., & Campbell, L. A. (2001b). Reliability of DSM-IV anxiety and mood disorders: implications for the classification of emotional disorders. *Journal of Abnormal Psychology, 110*, 49–58.

Brown, T. A., Moras, K., Zinbarg, R. E., & Barlow, D. H. (1993). Diagnostic and symptom distinguishability of generalized anxiety disorder and obsessive-compulsive disorder. *Behaviour Therapy, 24*, 227–240.

Buhr, K. & Dugas, M. J. (2002). The intolerance of uncertainty scale: psychometric properties of the English version. *Behaviour Research and Therapy, 40*, 931–945.

Buhr, K. & Dugas, M. J. (2006). Investigating the construct validity of intolerance of uncertainty and its unique relationship with worry. *Journal of Anxiety Disorders, 20*, 222–236.

Buhr, K. & Dugas, M. J. (2009). The role of fear of anxiety and intolerance of uncertainty in worry: an experimental manipulation. *Behaviour Research and Therapy*, *47*, 215–223.

Butler, G., Fennell, M., Robson, P., & Gelder, M. (1991). Comparison of behaviour therapy and cognitive behaviour therapy in the treatment of generalized anxiety disorder. *Journal of Consulting and Clinical Psychology, 59*, 167–175.

Carpenter, W. T., Bustillo, J. R., Thaker, G. K., van Os, J., Krueger, R. F., & Green, M. J. (2009). Psychoses: Cluster 3 of the proposed meta-structure for DSM-V and ICD-11. *Psychological Medicine, 39*, 2025–2042.

Carter, R. M., Wittchen, H.-U., Pfister, H., & Kessler, R. C. (2001). One-year prevalence of subthreshold and threshold DSM-IV generalized anxiety disorder in a nationally representative sample. *Depression and Anxiety, 13*, 78–88.

Chessick, C. A., Allen, M. H., Thase, M., Batista Miralha da Cunha, A. B., Kapczinski, F. F., de Lima, M. S., & dos Santos Souza, J. J. (2006). Azapirones for generalized anxiety disorder. *Cochrane Database Systematic Review, 3*, CD006115.

Christensen, H., Griffiths, K. M., Korten, A. E., Brittliffe, K., & Groves, C. (2004). A comparison of changes in anxiety and depression symptoms of spontaneous users and trial participants of a cognitive behaviour therapy website. *Journal of Medical Internet Research, 6*, e46.

Clarke, D. E., Narrow, W. E., Regier, D. A., Kuramoto, S. J., Kupfer, D. J., Kuhl, E. A., … Kraemer, H. C. (2013). DSM-5 Field Trials in the United States and Canada. Part I: Study design, sampling stratgy, implementation and analytic approaches. *American Journal of Psychiatry, 170*, 43–58.

Coles, M. E. & Heimberg, R. G. (2005). Thought control strategies in generalized anxiety disorder. *Cognitive Therapy and Research, 29*, 47–56.

Comer, J. S., Pincus, D. B., & Hofmann, S. G. (2012). Generalized anxiety disorder and the proposed associated symptoms criterion change for DSM-5 in a treatment-seeking sample of anxious youth. *Depression and Anxiety, 29*, 994–1003.

Covin, R., Ouimet, A. J., Seeds, P. M., & Dozois, D. J. A. (2008). A meta-analysis of CBT for pathological worry among clients with GAD. *Journal of Anxiety Disorders, 22*, 108–116.

Cox, B. J., Clara, I. P., & Enns, M. W. (2002). Posttraumatic stress disorder and the structure of common mental disorders. *Depression and Anxiety, 15*, 168–171.

Craigie, M. A., Rees, C., Marsh, A., & Nathan, P. (2008). Mindfulness-based cognitive therapy for generalized anxiety disorder: a preliminary evaluation. *Behavioural and Cognitive Psychotherapy, 36*, 553–568.

Craske, M. G., Barlow, D. H., & O'Leary, T. A. (1992). *Mastery of your anxiety and worry*. Albany, NY: Graywnd Publications.

Craske, M. G., Rapee, R. M., Jackel, L., & Barlow, D. H. (1989). Qualitative dimensions of worry in DSM-III-R generalized anxiety disorder subjects and non-anxious controls. *Behaviour Research and Therapy, 27*, 397–402.

Critchfield, K. L., Henry, W. P., Castonguay, L. G., & Borkovec, T. D. (2007). Interpersonal process and outcome in variants of cognitive-behavioural psychotherapy. *Journal of Clinical Psychiatry, 63*, 31–51.

Cuijpers, P., Sijbrandij, M., Koole, S., Huibers, M., Berking, M., & Andersson, G. (2014). Psychological treatment of generalized anxiety disorder: a meta-analysis. *Clinical Psychology Review, 34*, 130–140.

Davey, G. C., Hampton, J., Farrell, J., & Davidson, S. (1992). Some characteristics of worrying: evidence for worrying and anxiety as separate constructs. *Personality and Individual Differences, 13*, 133–147.

Davis, L., Barlow, D. H., & Smith, L. (2010). Comorbidity and the treatment of principal anxiety disorders in a naturalistic sample. *Behaviour Therapy, 41*, 296–305.

Davis, R. N. & Valentiner, D. P. (2000). Does meta-cognitive theory enhance our understanding of pathological worry and anxiety? *Personality and Individual Differences, 29*(3), 513–526.

Dayle Jones, K. (2012). A critique of the DSM-5 field trials. *Journal of Nervous and Mental Disease, 200*, 517–519.

De Jong-Meyer, R., Beck, B., & Riede, K. (2009). Relationships between rumination, worry, intolerance of uncertainty and metacognitive beliefs. *Personality and Individual Differences, 46*(4), 547–551.

Decker, M. L., Turk, C. L., Hess, B., & Murray, C. E. (2008). Emotion regulation among individuals classified with and without generalized anxiety disorder. *Journal of Anxiety Disorders, 22*, 485–494.

Di Nardo, P. A., Brown, T. A., & Barlow, D. H. (1994). *Anxiety disorders interview schedule for DSM-IV : lifetime version (ADIS-IV-L)*. New York, NY: Oxford University Press.

Di Nardo, P. A., Moras, K., Barlow, D. H., Rapee, R. M., & Brown, T. A. (1993). Reliability of DSM-III-R anxiety disorder categories: using the Anxiety Disorders Interview Schedule-Revised (ADIS-R). *Archives of General Psychiatry, 50*, 251–256.

Di Nardo, P. A., O'Brien, G. T., Waddell, M. T., & Blanchard, E. B. (1983). Reliability of DSM-III anxiety disorder categories using a new structured interview. *Archives of General Psychiatry, 40*, 1070–1074.

Donegan, E. & Dugas, M. J. (2012). Generalized anxiety disorder: a comparison of symptom change in adults receiving cognitive-behavioural therapy or applied relaxation. *Journal of Consulting and Clinical Psychology, 80*, 490–496.

Dugas, M. J., Brillon, P., Savard, P., Turcotte, J., Gaudet, A., Ladouceur, R., … Gervais, N. J. (2010). A randomized clinical trial of cognitive-behavioural therapy and applied relaxation for adults with generalized anxiety disorder. *Behaviour Therapy, 41*, 46–58.

Dugas, M. J., Francis, K., & Bouchard, S. (2009). Cognitive behavioural therapy and applied relaxation for generalized anxiety disorder: a time series analysis of change in worry and somatic anxiety. *Cognitive Behaviour Therapy, 38*, 29–41.

Dugas, M. J., Gagnon, F., Ladouceur, R., & Freeston, M. H. (1998). Generalized anxiety disorder: a preliminary test of a conceptual model. *Behaviour Research and Therapy, 36*, 215–226.

Dugas, M. J., Hedayati, M., Karavidas, A., Buhr, K., Francis, K., & Phillips, N. A. (2005). Intolerance of uncertainty and information processing: evidence of biased recall and interpretations. *Cognitive Therapy and Research, 29*, 57–70.

Dugas, M. J. & Ladouceur, R. (2000). Treatment of GAD: targeting intolerance of uncertainty in two types of worry. *Behaviour Modification, 24*, 635–657.

Dugas, M. J., Ladouceur, R., Leger, E., Freeston, M. H., Langlois, F., Provencher, M. D., & Boisvert, J. M. (2003). Group cognitive-behavioural therapy for generalized anxiety disorder: treatment outcome and long-term follow-up. *Journal of Consulting and Clinical Psychology, 71*, 821–825.

Dupuy, J. -B., Beudoin, S., Rheaume, J., Ladouceur, R., & Dugas, M. J. (2001). Worry: daily self-report in clinical and non-clinical populations. *Behaviour Research and Therapy, 39*, 1249–1255.

Eaton, N. R., Keyes, K. M., Krueger, R. F., Noordhof, A., Skodol, A. E., Markon, K. E., … Hasin, D. S. (2012). Ethnicity and psychiatric comorbidity in a national sample: evidence for latent comorbidity factor invariance and connections with disorder prevalence. *Social Psychiatry and Psychiatric Epidemiology, 48*, 701–710.

Eaton, N. R., Krueger, R. F., & Oltmanns, T. F. (2011). Aging and the structure and long-term stability of the internalizing spectrum of personality and psychopathology. *Psychology and Aging, 26*, 987–993.

Erickson, D. H. (2003). Group cognitive behavioural therapy for heterogeneous anxiety disorders. *Cognitive Behaviour Therapy, 32*, 179–186.

Erickson, D. H., Janeck, A., & Tallman, K. (2007). Group cognitive-behavioural group for patients with various anxiety disorders. *Psychiatric Services, 58*, 1205–1211.

Evans, S., Ferrando, S., Findler, M., Stowell, C., Smart, C., & Haglin, D. (2008). Mindfulness-based cognitive therapy for generalized anxiety disorder. *Journal of Anxiety Disorders, 22*, 716–721.

Farchione, T. J., Fairholme, C. P., Ellard, K. K., Boisseau, C. L, Thompson-Hollands, J., Carl, J. R., … Barlow, D. H. (2012). Unified protocol for transdiagnostic treatment of emotional disorders: a randomized controlled trial. *Behaviour Therapy, 43*, 666–678.

Fergusson, D. M., Horwood, L. J., & Boden, J. M. (2006). Structure of internalizing symptoms in early adulthood. *British Journal of Psychiatry, 189*, 540–546.

First, M. B., Spitzer, R. L., Gibbon, M., & Williams, J. B. W. (1997). *Structured Clinical Interview for DSM-IV Axis I disorders (SCID I)*. New York, NY: Biometric Research Department.

Fisher, P. L. (2006). The efficacy of psychological treatments for generalized anxiety disorder. In G. C. Davey & A. Wells (Eds.), *Worry and its psychological disorders:theory, assessment and treatment.* West Sussex, England: John Wiley & Sons.

Fisher, P. L. & Durham, R. C. (1999). Recovery rates in generalized anxiety disorder following psychological therapy: an analysis of clinically significant change in the STAI-T across outcome studies since 1990. *Psychological Medicine, 29*(6), 1425–1434.

Foa, E. B. & Kozak, M. J. (1986). Emotional processing of fear: exposure to corrective information. *Psychological Bulletin, 99*(1), 20–35.

Fresco, D. M., Mennin, D. S., Heimberg, R. G., & Ritter, M. (2013). Emotion regulation therapy for generalized anxiety disorder. *Cognitive and Behavioural Practice, 20*, 282–300.

Friborg, O., Martinussen, M., Kaiser, S., Overgard, K. T., & Rosenvinge, J. H. (2013). Comorbidity of personality disorders in anxiety disorders: a meta-analysis of 30 years of research. *Journal of Affective Disorders, 145*, 143–155.

Furer, P., Walker, J. R., & Stein, M. B. (2007). *Treating health anxiety and fear of death: a practitioner's guide.* New York, NY: Springer.

Garfinkle, E. J. & Behar, E. (2012). Advances in psychotherapy for generalized anxiety disorder. *Current Psychiatric Reports, 14*, 203–210.

Gentes, E. L. & Ruscio, A. M. (2011). A meta-analysis of the relation of intolerance of uncertainty to symptoms of generalized anxiety disorder, major depressive disorder, and obsessive-compulsive disorder. *Clinical Psychology Review, 31*, 923–933.

Glenn, C. R. & Klonsky, E. D. (2009). Emotion dysregulation as a core feature of borderline personality disorder. *Journal of Personality Disorders, 23*, 20–28.

Goldberg, D. P., Andrews, G., Krueger, R., & Hobbs, M. J. (2009). Emotional disorders: cluster 4 of the proposed meta-structure for DSM-V. *Psychological Medicine, 39*, 2043–2059.

Goldman, N., Dugas, M. J., Sexton, K. A., & Gervais, N. J. (2007). The impact of written exposure on worry: a preliminary investigation. *Behaviour Modification, 31*, 512–538.

Goncalves, D. C. & Byrne, G. J. (2012). Interventions for generalized anxiety disorder in older adults: systematic review and meta-analysis. *Journal of Anxiety Disorders, 26*, 1–11.

Gotzsche, P. C. (2014). Why I think antidepressants cause more harm than good. *The Lancet/Psychiatry, 1*, 104–106.

Gould, R. A., Otto, M. W., Pollack, M. H., & Yap, L. . (1997). Cognitive behavioural and pharmacological treatment of generalized anxiety disorder: a preliminary meta-analysis. *Behaviour Therapy, 28*, 285–305.

Grant, B. F., Hasin, D., Stinson, F. S., Dawson, D. A., Ruan, W. J., Goldstein, R. B., ... Huang, B. (2005). Prevalence, correlates, co-morbidity, and comparative disability of DSM-IV generalized anxiety disorder in the

USA: results from the National Epidemiologic Survey on Alcohol and Related Conditions. *Psychological Medicine, 35,* 1747–1759.

Gratz, K. L. & Roemer, E. (2004). Multidimensional assessment of emotion regulation and dysregulation: development, factor structure, and initial validation of the difficulties in emotion regulation scale. *Journal of Psychopathology and Behavioural Assessment, 26,* 41–54.

Green, J. G., McLaughlin, K. A., Berglund, P. A., Gruber, M. J., Sampson, N. A., Zaslavsky, A. M., & Kessler, R. C. (2010). Childhood adversities and adult psychiatric disorders in the national comorbidity survey replication I: associations with first onset of DSM-IV disorders. *Archives of General Psychiatry, 67,* 113–123.

Hanrahan, F., Field, A. P., Jones, F. W., & Davey, G. C. L. (2013). A meta-analysis of cognitive therapy for worry in generalized anxiety disorder. *Clinical Psychology Review, 33,* 120–132.

Harvey, A. G., Watkins, E. R., Mansell, W., & Shafran, R. (2004). *Cognitive behavioural processes across psychological disorders: a transdiagnostic approach to reseach and treatment.* Oxford, UK: Oxford University Press.

Hayes, S. C., Wilson, K. G., Gifford, E. V., Follette, V. M., & Strosahl, K. (1996). Experiential avoidance and behavioural disorders: a functional dimensional approach to diagnosis and treatment. *Journal of Consulting and Clinical Psychology, 64,* 1152–1168.

Hayes-Skelton, S. A., Orsillo, S. M., & Roemer, L. (2013). An acceptance-based behavioural therapy for individuals with generalized anxiety disorder. *Cognitive and Behavioural Practice, 20,* 264–281.

Hayes-Skelton, S. A., Roemer, L., & Orsillo, S. M. (2013). A randomized clinical trial comparing an acceptance-based behaviour therapy to applied relaxation for generalized anxiety disorder. *Journal of Consulting and Clinical Psychology, 81,* 761–773.

Hebert, E. A., Dugas, M. J., Tulloch T. G., & Holowka, D. W. (2014). Positive beliefs about worry: a psychometric evaluation of the Why Worry-II. *Personality and Individual Differences, 56,* 3–8.

Herring, M. P., Jacob, . L., Suveg, C., Dishman, R. K., & O'connor, P. J. (2012). Feasibility of exercise training for the short-term treatment of generalized anxiety disorder: a randomized controlled trial. *Psychotherapy and Psychosomatics, 81,* 21–28.

Hettema, J. M., Neale, M. C., & Kendler, K. S. (2001). A review and meta-analysis of the genetic epidemiology of anxiety disorders. *American Journal of Psychiatry, 158,* 1568–1578.

Hettema, J. M., Neale, M. C., Myers, J. M., Prescott, C. A., & Kendler, K. S. (2006). A population-based twin study of the relationship between neuroticism and internalizing disorders. *American Journal of Psychiatry, 163,* 857–864.

Hettema, J. M., Prescott, C. A., & Kendler, K. S. (2003). The effects of anxiety, substance use, and conduct disorders on the risk of major depressive disorder. *Psychological Medicine, 33,* 1423–1432.

Hettema, J. M., Prescott, C. A., & Kendler, K. S. (2004). Genetic and environmental sources of covariation between generalized anxiety disorder and neuroticism. *American Journal of Psychiatry, 161,* 1581–1587.

Hjemdal, O., Hagen, R., Nordahl, H. M., & Wells, A. (2013). Metacognitive therapy for generalized anxiety disorder: nature, evidence and an individual case illustration. *Cognitive and Behavioural Practice, 20,* 301–313.

Hidalgo, R. B., Tupler, L. A., & Davidson, J. R. (2007). An effect-size analysis of pharmacologic treatments for generalized anxiety disorder. *Journal of Psychopharmacology, 21,* 864–872.

Hofmann, S. G., Moscovitch, D. A., Litz, B. T., Kim, H. J., Davis, L. L., & Pizzagalli, D. A. (2005). The worried mind: autonomic and prefrontal activation during worrying. *Emotion, 5,* 464–475.

Hofmann, S.G. & Smits, J.A.J. (2008). Cognitive-behavioural therapy for adult anxiety disorders: a meta-analysis of randomized placebo-controlled trials. *Journal of Clinical Psychiatry, 69,* 621–632.

Hoge, E. A., Bui, E., Marques, L., Metcalf, C. A., Morris, L. K., Robinaugh, D. J., ... Simon, N. M. (2013). Randomized controlled trial of mindfulness meditation for generalized anxiety disorder: effects on anxiety and stress reactivity. *Journal of Clinical Psychiatry, 74,* 786–792.

Hoyer, J., Becker, E. S., & Roth, W. T. (2001). Characteristics of worry in GAD patients, social phobics and controls. *Depression and Anxiety, 13,* 89–96.

Hoyer, J., Beesdo, K., Gloster, A. T., Runge, J., Hofler, M., & Becker, E. S. (2009). Worry exposure versus applied relaxation in the treatment of generalized anxiety disorder. *Psychotherapy and Psychosomatics, 78,* 106–115.

Hunot, V., Churchill, R., Silva de Lima, M., & Teixeira, V. (2007). Psychological therapies for generalized anxiety disorder. *Cochrane Database of Systematic Reviews, 1,* CD001848.

Hunot, V., Churchill, R., Teixeira, V., & Silva de Lima, M. (2010). Psychological therapies for people with generalized anxiety disorder. *Cochrane Database of Systematic Reviews, 4,* CD001848.

Hunt, C., Issakidis, C., & Andrews, G. (2002). DSM-IV generalized anxiety disorder in the Australian National Survey of Mental Health and Well-Being. *Psychological Medicine, 32,* 649–659.

Hyman, S. E. (2007). Can neuroscience be integrated into the DSM-V? *Nature Reviews: Neuroscience, 8,* 725–732.

Jackson, J. S., Torres, M., Caldwell, C. H., Neighbors, H. W., Nesse, R. M., Taylor, R. J., ... Williams, D. R. (2004). The National Survey of American Life: a study of racial, ethnis and cultural influences on mental disorders and mental health. *International Journal of Methods in Psychiatric Research, 13,* 196–207.

Johansson, R. & Andersson, G. (2012). Internet-based psychological treatments for depression. *Expert Review of Neurotherapeutics, 12*, 861–869.

Johnston, L., Titov, N., Andrews, G., Spence, J., & Dear, B.F. (2011). A RCT of a transdiagnostic internet-delivered treatment for three anxiety disorders: examination of support roles and disorder-specific outcomes. *PLoS One, 6*(11), e28079.

Judd, L. L., Akiskal, H. S., Maser, J. D., Zeller, P. J., Endicott, J., Coryell, W., ... Keller, M. B. (1998). A prospective 12-year study of subsyndromal and syndromal depressive symptoms in unipolar major depressive disorders. *Archives of General Psychiatry, 55*, 694–700.

Kagan, J. & Snidman, N. (1999). Early childhood predictors of adult anxiety disorders. *Biological Psychiatry, 46*, 1536–1541.

Kendell, R. E. & Jablensky, A. (2003). Distinguishing the validity and utility of psychiatric diagnoses. *American Journal of Psychiatry, 160*, 4–12.

Kendler, K. S., Aggen, S. H., Knudsen, G. P., Røysamb, E., Neale, M. C., & Reichborn-Kjeennerud, T. (2011). The structure of genetic and environmental risk factors for syndromal and subsyndromal common DSM-IV Axis I and Axis II disorders. *American Journal of Psychiatry, 168*, 29–39.

Kendler, K. S., Davis, C. G., & Kessler, R. C. (1997). The familial aggregation of common psychiatric and substance use disorders in the National Comorbidity Survey: a family history study. *British Journal of Psychiatry, 170*, 541–548.

Kendler, K. S., Gardner, C. O., Gatz, M., & Pedersen, N. L. (2007). The sources of co-morbidity between major depression and generalized anxiety disorder in a Swedish national twin sample. *Psychological Medicine, 37*, 453–462.

Kendler, K. S., Neale, M. C., Kessler, R. C., Heath, A. C., & Eaves, L. J. (1992). Generalized anxiety disorder in women. A population-based twin study. *Archives of General Psychiatry, 49*, 267–272.

Kendler, K. S., Neale, M. C., Kessler, R. C., Heath, A. C., & Eaves, L. J. (1994). Clinical characteristics of familial generalized anxiety disorder. *Anxiety, 1*, 186–191.

Kendler, K. S., Prescott, C. A., Myers, J. M., & Neale, M. C. (2003). The structure of genetic and environmental risk factors for common psychiatric and substance use disorders in men and women. *Archives of General Psychiatry, 60*, 929–937.

Kendler, K. S., Walters, E. E., Neale, M. C., Heath, A. C., & Eaves, L. J. (1995). The structure of the genetic and environmental risk factors for six major psychiatric disorders in women: phobia, generalized anxiety disorder, panic disorder, bulimia, major depression and alcoholism. *Archives of General Psychiatry, 52*, 374–383.

Kerns, C. E., Mennin, D. S., Farach, F. J., & Nocera, C. C. (2014). Utilizing an ability-based measure to detect emotion regulation deficits in generalized anxiety disorder. *Journal of Psychopathology and Behavioural Assessment, 36*, 115–123.

Kessler, R. C., Avenevoli, S., Costello, E. J., Georgiades, K., Green, J., Gruber, M. J., ... Merikangas, K. R. (2012a). Prevalence, persistence, and socoidemographic correlates of DSM-IV disorders in the National Comorbidity Survey Replication Adolescent Supplement. *Archives of General Psychiatry, 69,* 372–380.

Kessler, R. C., Avenevoli, S., Costello, E. J., Green, J. G., Gruber, M. J., Heeringa, S., ... Zaslavsky, A. M. (2009). Design and field procedures in the US National Comorbidity Survey Replication Adolescent Supplement (NCS-A). *International Journal of Methods in Psychiatric Research, 18,* 69–83.

Kessler, R. C., Avenevoli, S., McLaughlin, K. A., Green, J., Lakoma, M. D., Petukhova, M., ... Merikangas, K. R. (2012b). Lifetime co-morbidity of DSM-IV disorders in the US National Comorbidity Survey Replication Adolescent Supplement (NCS-A). *Psychological Medicine, 42,* 1997–2010.

Kessler, R. C., Berglund, P. A., Dewit, D. J., Üstun, T. B., Wang, P. S., & Wittchen, H. -U. (2002). Distinguishing generalized anxiety disorder from major depression: prevalence and impairment from current pure and comorbid disorders in the US and Ontario. *International Journal of Methods in Psychiatric Research, 11,* 99–111.

Kessler, R. C., Berglund, P., Demler, O. V., Jin, R., Merikangas, K. R., & Walters, E. E. (2005b). Lifetime prevalence and age-of-onset distributions of DSM-IV disorders in the national comorbidity replication. *Archives of General Psychiatry, 62,* 593–602.

Kessler, R. C., Brandenburg, N., Lane, M., Roy-Byrne, P., Stang, P., Stein, D. J., & Wittchen, H. -U. (2005c). Rethinking the duration requirement for generalized anxiety disorder: evidence from the National Comorbidity Survey Replication. *Psychological Medicine, 35,* 1073–1082.

Kessler, R. C., Haro, J. M., Heeringa, S. G., Pennell, B. -E., & Üstun, T. B. (2006). The World Health Organization world mental health survey initiative. *Epidemiologia e Psichiatria Sociale 15,* 161–166.

Kessler, R. C. & Merikangas, K. R. (2004). The National Comorbidity Survey Replication (NCS-R): background and aims. *International Journal of Methods in Psychiatric Research 13,* 60–68.

Kessler, R. C. & Üstun, T. B. (2004). The World Mental Health (WMH) Survey Initiative Version of the World Health Organization (WHO) Composite International Diagnostic Interview (CIDI). *International Journal of Methods in Psychiatric Research, 13,* 93–121.

Kessler, R. C., Wai, T. C., Demler, O. V., Merikangas, K. R., & Walters, E. E. (2005a). Prevalence, severity, and comorbidity of 12-month DSM-IV disorders in the National Survey Replication. *Archives of General Psychiatry, 62,* 617–627.

Kessler, R. C. & Wittchen, H. -U. (2002). Patterns and correlates of generalized anxiety disorder in community samples. *Journal of Clinical Psychiatry, 63*(Suppl. 8), S4–S10.

Kessler, R. C., Wittchen, H. -U., Abelson, J. M., McGonagle, K. A., Schwarz, N., Kendler, K. S., ... Zhao, S. (1998). Methodological studies of the Composite

International Diagnostic Interview (CIDI) in the US National Comorbidity Survey. *International Journal of Methods in Psychiatric Research, 7*, 33–55.

Krueger, R. F. (1999a). Personality traits in late adolescence predict mental disorders in early adulthood: A prospective-epidemiological study. *Journal of Personality, 67*, 39–65.

Krueger, R. F. (1999b). The structure of common mental disorders. *Archives of General Psychiatry, 56*, 921–926.

Krueger, R. F., Caspi, A., Moffitt, T. E., & Silva, P. A. (1998). The structure and stability of common mental disorders (DSM-III-R): a longitudinal-epidemiological study. *Journal of Abnormal Psychology, 107*, 216–227.

Krueger, R. F., Chentsova-Dutton, Y. E., Markon, K. E., Goldberg, D. P., & Ormel, J. (2003). A cross-cultural study of the structure of comorbidity among common psychopathological syndromes in the general health care setting. *Journal of Abnormal Psychology, 107*, 216–227.

Krueger, R. F., & Markon, K. E. (2006). Reinterpreting comorbidity: A model-based approach to understanding and classifying psychopathology. *Annual Review of Clinical Psychology, 2*, 111–133.

Krueger, R. F. & South, S. C. (2009). Externalizing disorders: cluster 5 of the proposed meta-structure for DSM-V and ICD-11. *Psychological Medicine, 39*, 2061–2070.

Ladouceur, R., Blais, F., Freeston, M. H., & Dugas, M. J. (1998). Problem solving and problem orientation in generalized anxiety disorder. *Journal of Anxiety Disorders, 12*, 139–152.

Ladouceur, R., Dugas, M. J., Freeston, M. H., Leger, E., Gagnon, F., & Thibodeau, N. (2000). Efficacy of a cognitive-behavioural treatment for generalized anxiety disorder: evaluation in a controlled clinical trial. *Journal of Consulting and Clinical Psychology, 68*, 957–964.

Ladouceur, R., Gosselin, P., & Dugas, M. J. (2000). Experimental manipulation of intolerance of uncertainty: a study of a theoretical model of worry. *Behaviour Research and Therapy, 38*, 933–941.

Ladouceur, R., Talbot, F., & Dugas, M. J. (1997). Behavioural expressions of intolerance of uncertainty in worry: experimental findings. *Behaviour Modification, 21*, 355–371.

Lahey, B. B., Rathouz, P. J., van Hulle, C., Urbano, R. C., Krueger, R. F., Applegate, B., … Waldman, I. D. (2008). Testing structural models of DSM-IV symptoms of common forms of child and adolescent psychopathology. *Journal of Abnormal Child Psychology 36*, 187–206.

LaLonde, C. D. & Van Lieshout, R. J. (2011). Treating generalized anxiety disorder with second generation antipsychotics: a systematic review and meta-analysis. *Journal of Clinical Psychopharmacology, 31*, 326–333.

Lampe, L. (2004). *Take control of your worry: managing generalized anxiety disorder.* Sydney, AU: Simon & Schuster.

Laugesen, N., Dugas, M. J., & Bukowski, W. M. (2003). Understanding adolescent worry: the application of a cognitive model. *Journal of Abnormal Child Psychology, 31,* 55–64.

Laurens, K. R., Hobbs, M. J., Sunderland, M., Green, M. J., & Mould, G. L. (2012). Psychotic-like experiences in a community sample of 8,000 children aged 9 to 11 years: an item response theory analysis. *Psychological Medicine, 42,* 1495–1506.

Lee, J. K., Orsillo, S. M., Roemer, L., & Allen, L. B. (2010). Distress and avoidance in generalized anxiety disorder: exploring the relationships with intolerance of uncertainty and worry. *Cognitive Behaviour Therapy, 39,* 126–136.

Lee, S., Tsang, A., Ruscio, A. M., Haro, J. M., Stein, D. J., Alonso, J., ... Kessler, R. C. (2009). Implications of modifying the duration requirement of generalized anxiety disorder in developed and developing countries. *Psychological Medicine, 39,* 1163–1176.

Leichsenring, F., Salzer, S., Jaeger, U., Kachele, H., Kreische, R., Leweke, F., ... Leibing, E. (2009). Short-term psychodynamic psychotherapy and cognitive-behavioural therapy in generalized anxiety disorder: a randomized, controlled trial. *American Journal of Psychiatry, 166,* 875–881.

Llera, S. J. & Newman, M. G. (2010). Effects of worry on physiological and subjective reactivity to emotional stimuli in generalized anxiety disorder and nonanxious control participants. *Emotion, 10,* 640–650.

Lobbestael, J., Leurgans, M., & Arntz, A. (2011). Inter-rater reliability of the Structured Clinical Interview for DSM-IV Aixs I Disorders (SCID I) and Axis II Disorders (SCID II). *Clinical Psychology and Psychotherapy, 18,* 75–79.

Lumpkin, P. W., Silverman, W. K., Weems, C. F., Markham, M. R., & Kurtines, W. M. (2002). Treating a heterogeneous set of anxiety disorders in youth with group cognitive behavioural therapy: a partially nonconcurrent multiple-baseline evaluation. *Behaviour Therapy, 33,* 163–177.

Lyonfields, J. D., Borkovec, T. D., & Thayer, J. F. (1995). Vagal tone in generalized anxiety disorder and the effects of aversive imagery and worrisome thinking. *Behaviour Therapy, 26,* 457–466.

National Institute of Clinical Excellence, National Collaborating Centre for Mental Health (2011). *Generalised anxiety disorder in adults: management in primary, secondary and community care. NICE Clinical Guidelines, No. 113.* Leicester, UK: British Psychological Society.

Mahoney, A. & McEvoy, P. M. (2012a). A transdiagnostic examination of intolerance of uncertainty across anxiety and depressive disorders. *Cognitive Behaviour Therapy, 41,* 212–222.

Mahoney, A. & McEvoy, P. M. (2012b). Trait versus situation-specific intolerance of uncertainty in a clinical sample with anxiety and depressive disorders. *Cognitive Behaviour Therapy, 41,* 26–39.

Mahoney, A. & McEvoy, P. M. (2012c). Changes in intolerance of uncertainty during cognitive behaviour group therapy for social phobia. *Journal of Behaviour Therapy and Experimental Psychiatry, 43,* 849–854.

Maier, W., Gänsicke, M., Freyberger, H. J., Linz, M., Heun, R., & Lecrubier, Y. (2000). Generalized anxiety disorder (ICD-10) in primary care from a cross-cultural perspective: a valid diagnostic entity? *Acta Psychiatrica Scandinavica, 101*, 29–36.

Mannuzza, S., Fyer, A. J., Martin, M. S., Gallops, M. S., Endicott, J., Gorman, J. M., … Klein, D. F. (1989). Reliability of anxiety assessment, I: Diagnostic agreement. *Archives of General Psychiatry, 46*, 1093–1101.

Markon, K. E. (2010). Modeling psychopathology structure: A symptom-level analysis of Axis I and II disorders. *Psychological Medicine, 40*, 273–288.

Martin, J. L., Sainz-Pardo, M., Furukawa, T. A., Martin-Sanchez, E., Seoane, T., & Galan, C. (2007). Benzodiazepines in generalized anxiety disorder: heterogeneity of outcomes based on a systematic review and meta-analysis of clinical trials. *Journal of Psychopharmacology, 21*, 774–782.

Martinsen, E. W., Hoffart, A., & Solberg, Y. (1989). Aerobic and non-aerobic forms of exercise in the treatment of anxiety disorders. *Stress and Health, 5*, 115–120.

Maser, J. D., & Patterson, T. (2002). Spectrum and nosology: Implications for DSM-V Psychiatric *Clinics of North America, 25*, 855–885.

Matthews, A. & MacLeod, C. (1986). Discrimination of threat cues without awareness in anxiety states. *Journal of Abnormal Psychology, 95*, 131–138.

Mayo-Wilson, E. & Montgomery, P. (2013). Media-delivered cognitive behavioural therapy and behavioural therapy (self-help) for anxiety disorders in adults. *Cochrane Database of Systematic Reviews, 9*, CD005330.

McEvoy, P. M., Grove, R., & Slade, T. (2011). Epidemiology of anxiety disorders in the Australian general population: findings of the 2007 Australian National Survey of Mental Health and Wellbeing. *Australian and New Zealand Journal of Psychiatry, 45*, 957–967.

McEvoy, P. M. & Mahoney, A. E. J. (2011). Achieving certainty about the structure of intolerance of uncertainty in a treatment-seeking sample with anxiety and depression. *Journal of Anxiety Disorders, 25*, 112–122.

McEvoy, P. M. & Mahoney, A. E. J. (2012). To be sure, to be sure: intolerance of uncertainty mediates symptoms of various anxiety disorders and depression. *Behaviour Therapy, 43*, 533–545.

McEvoy, P. M. & Nathan, P. (2007). Effectiveness of cognitive behaviour therapy for diagnostically heterogeneous groups: a benchmarking study. *Journal of Consulting and Clinical Psychology, 75*, 344–350.

McLaughlin, K. A., Green, J. G., Gruber, M. J., Sampson, N. A., Zaslavsky, A. M., & Kessler, R. C. (2010). Childhood adversities and adult psychiatric disorders in the National Comorbidity Survey Replication II: Associations with persistence of DSM-IV disorders. *Archives of General Psychiatry, 67*, 124–132.

Mennin, D. S. & Fresco, D. M. (2011). *Emotion regulation therapy for complex and refractory presentations of anxiety and depression.* Paper presented at the Association for Behavioural and Cognitive Therapies, Toronto, Ontario.

Mennin, D. S., Fresco, D. M., & Aldao, A. (2012). *Increasing vagal flexibility predicts improved clinical outcomes in emotion regulation therapy for GAD.* Paper presented at the Association for Behavioural and Cognitive Therapies, National Harbor, MD.

Mennin, D. S., Fresco, D. M., Heimberg, R. G., & Ciesla, J. (2012). *Randomized control trial of emotion regulation therapy for generalized anxiety disorder and comorbid depression.* Paper presented at the Anxiety Disorders Association of America, Arlington, VA.

Mennin, D. S., Heimberg, R. G., Turk, C. L., & Fresco, D. M. (2002). Applying an emotion regulation framework to integrative approaches to generalized anxiety disorder. *Clinical Psychology: Science and Practice, 9*, 85–90.

Mennin, D. S., Heimberg, R. G., Turk, C. L., & Fresco, D. M. (2005). Preliminary evidence for an emotion dysregulation model of generalized anxiety disorder. *Behaviour Research and Therapy, 43*, 1281–1310.

Mennin, D. S., Holaway, R. M., Fresco, D. M., Moore, M. T., & Heimberg, R. G. (2007). Delineating components of emotion and its dysregulation in anxiety and mood psychopathology. *Behaviour Therapy, 38*, 284–301.

Merom, D., Phongsavan, P., Wagner, R., Chey, T., Marnane, C., Steel, Z., … Bauman, A. (2008). Promoting walking as an adjunct intervention to group cognitive behavioural therapy for anxiety disorders: a pilot group randomized trial. *Journal of Anxiety Disorders, 6*, 959–968.

Mewton, L., Wong, N., & Andrews, G. (2012). The effectiveness of internet cognitive behavioural therapy for generalized anxiety disorder in clinical practice. *Depression and Anxiety, 29*, 843–849.

Meyer, T. J., Miller, M. L., Metzger, R. L., & Borkovec, T. D. (1990). Development and validation of the Penn State Worry Questionnaire. *Behaviour Research and Therapy, 28*, 487–495.

Michelson, S. E., Lee, J. K., Orsillo, S. M., & Roemer, L. (2011). The role of values-consistent behaviour in generalized anxiety disorder. *Depression and Anxiety, 28*, 358–366.

Mitte, K. (2005). A meta-analysis of the efficacy of psycho- and pharmacotherapy in panic disorder with and without agoraphobia. *Journal of Affective Disorders, 88*, 27–45.

Mitte, K., Noack, P., Steil, R., & Hautzinger, M. (2005). A meta-analytic review of the efficacy of drug treatment in generalized anxiety disorder. *Journal of Clinical Psychopharmacology, 25*, 141–150.

Moffitt, T. E., Harrington, H. L., Capsi, A., Kim-Cohen, J., Goldberg, D. P., Gregory, A., & Poulton, R. (2007). Depression and generalized anxiety disorder: cumulative and sequential comorbidity in a birth cohort followed to age 32. *Archives of General Psychiatry, 64*, 651–660.

Molina, S. & Borkovec, T. D. (1994). The Penn State Worry Questionnaire: psychometric properties and associated characteristics. In G. C. L. Davey & F. Tallis (Eds.), *Worrying: perspectives on theory, assessment and treatment* (pp. 265–283). New York, NY: Wiley.

Mooney, K. & Padesky, C. A. (2000). Applying client creativity to recurrent problems: constructing possibilities and tolerating doubt. *Journal of Cognitive
Psychotherapy, 14,* 149–161.

Morgan, L. P. K., Graham, J. R., Hayes-Skelton, S. A., Orsillo, S. M., & Roemer, L.
(2014). Relationships between amount of post-intervention mindfulness practice
and follow-up outcome variables in an acceptance-based behaviour therapy for
generalized anxiety disorder: the importance of informal practice. *Journal of
Contextual Behavioural Science, 3,* 173–178.

Myers, S. G. & Wells, A. (2013). An experimental manipulation of metacognition: a
test of the metacognitive model of obsessive-compulsive symptoms. *Behaviour
Research and Therapy, 51,* 177–184.

National Collaborating Center for Mental Health (2011). *Generalized anxiety disorder in adults: management in primary, secondary, and community
care.* London: The British Psychological Society and The Royal College of
Psychiatrists.

Newby, J. M., Mackenzie, A., Williams, A. D., McIntyre, K., Watts, S., Wong, N., &
Andrews, G. (2013). Internet cognitive behavioural therapy for mixed anxiety
and depression: a randomized controlled trial and evidence of efffectiveness in
primary care. *Psychological Medicine,* 1–14.

Newby, J. M, Mewton, L., Williams, A. D., & Andrews, G. (2014). Effectiveness of
transdiagnostic internet cognitive behavioural treatment for mixed anxiety and
depression in primary care. *Journal of Affective Disorders, 165,* 45–52.

Newman, M. G., Castonguay, L. G., Borkovec, T. D., Fisher, A. J., Boswell, J. F.,
Szkodny, L. E., & Nordberg, S. S. (2011). A randomized controlled trial of
cognitive-behavioural therapy for generalized anxiety disorder with integrated
techniques from emotion-focused and interpersonal therapies. *Journal of
Consulting and Clinical Psychology, 79,* 171–181.

Newman, M. G., Castonguay, L. G., Borkovec, T. D., Fisher, A. J., & Nordberg, S. S.
(2008b). An open trial of integrative therapy for generalized anxiety disorder.
Psychotherapy, 45, 135–147.

Newman, M. G., Castonguay, L. G., Fisher, A. J., & Borkovec, T. D. (2008a). The
addition of interpersonal and emotional processing techniques to the treatment of generalized anxiety disorder. In: C. T. Taylor & N. Amir (Chairs), *Novel
approaches to the treatment of generalized anxiety disorder.* Paper presented at the
42nd Annual Meeting of the Association for the Advancement of Behavioural and
Cognitive Therapies, November 2008, Orlando, FL.

Newman, M. G. & Fisher, A. J. (2013). Mediated moderation in combined cognitive
behavioural therapy versus component treatments for generalized anxiety disorder. *Journal of Consulting and Clinical Psychology, 81,* 405–414.

Newman, M. G. & Llera, S. J. (2011). A novel theory of experiential avoidance in
generalized anxiety disorder: a review and synthesis of research supporting a
contrast avoidance model of worry. *Clinical Psychology Review, 31,* 371–382.

Newman, M. G., Przeworski, A., Fishler, A. J., & Borkovec, T. D. (2010). Diagnostic comorbidity in adults with generalized anxiety disorder: impact of comorbidity on psychotherapy outcome and impact of psychotherapy on comorbid diagnoses. *Behaviour Therapy, 41,* 59–72.

Norton, P. J. (2012a). *Group cognitive behavioural therapy of anxiety: a transdiagnostic treatment manual.* New York, NY: Guilford Press.

Norton, P. J. (2012b). A randomized clinical trial of transdiagnostic cognitive-behavioural treatments for anxiety disorders by comparison to relaxation training. *Behaviour Therapy, 43,* 506–517.

Norton, P. J., Barrera, T. L., Mathew, A. R., Chamberlain, L. D., Szafranski, D. D., Reddy, R., & Smith, A. H. (2013). Effect of transdiagnostic CBT for anxiety disorders on comorbid diagnoses. *Depression and Anxiety, 30,* 168–173.

Norton, P. J. & Hope, D.A. (2002). *Anxiety treatment program: therapist manual.* Unpublished treatment manual.

Norton, P. J. & Philipp, L. M. (2008). Transdiagnostic approaches to the treatment of anxiety disorders: a meta-analytic review. *Psychotherapy: Theory, Research, Practice, and Training, 45,* 214–226.

Novick-Kline, P., Turk, C. L., Mennin, D. S., Hoyt, E. A., & Gallagher, C. L. (2005). Level of emotional awareness as a differentiating variable between individuals with and without generalized anxiety disorder. *Journal of Anxiety Disorders, 19,* 557–572.

Ost, L.-G. (1987). Applied relaxation: description of a coping technique and review of controlled studies. *Behaviour Research and Therapy, 25,* 397–409.

Padesky, C. A. (1993). *Socratic questioning: changing minds or guiding discovery?* Paper presented at the keynote address at the European Congress of Behavioural and Cognitive Therapies, London.

Padesky, C. A. (1994). Schema change processes in cognitive therapy. *Clinical Psychology and Psychotherapy, 1,* 267–278.

Papageorgiou, C. & Wells, A. (1999). Process and meta-cognitive dimensions of depressive and anxious thoughts and relationships with emotional intensity. *Clinical Psychology and Psychotherapy, 6,* 156–162.

Paxling, B., Almlov, J., Dahlin, M., Carlbring, P., Breitholtz, E., Eriksson, T., & Andersson, G. (2011). Guided internet-delivered cognitive behaviour therapy for generalized anxiety disorder: a randomized controlled trial. *Cognitive Behaviour Therapy, 40,* 159–173.

Peasley-Miklus, C. & Vrana, S. R. (2000). Effect of worrisome and relaxing thinking on fearful emotional processing. *Behaviour Research and Therapy, 38,* 129–144.

Penney, A. M., Mazmanian, D., & Rudanycz, C. (2013). Comparing positive and negative beliefs about worry in predicting generalized anxiety disorder symptoms. *Canadian Journal of Behavioural Science, 45,* 34–41.

Pine, D. S., Cohen, P., Gurley, D., Brook, J., & Ma, Y. (1998). The risk for early adulthood anxiety and depressive disorders in adolescents with anxiety and depressive disorders. *Archives of General Psychiatry, 55,* 56–64.

Provencher, M. D., Dugas, M. J., & Ladouceur, R. (2004). Efficacy of problem-solving training and cognitive exposure in the treatment of generalized anxiety disorder: a case replication series. *Cognitive and Behavioural Practice, 11*, 404–414.

Rapee, R. M. (1991). Generalized anxiety disorder: a review of clinical features and theoretical concepts. *Clinical Psychology Review, 11*, 419–440.

Regier, D. A., Kuhl, E. A., & Kupfer, D. J. (2013). The DSM-5: classification and criteria change. *World Psychiatry, 12*, 92–98.

Regier, D. A., Narrow, W. E., Clark, D. E., Kraemer, H. C., Kuramoto, S. J., Kuhl, E. A., & Kupfer, D. J. (2013). DSM-5 Field Trials in the United States and Canada, Part III: Test–retest reliability of selected categorical diagnoses. *American Journal of Psychiatry, 170*, 71–82.

Regier, D. A., Narrow, W. E., Kuhl, W. E., & Kupfer, D. J. (2009). The conceptual development of DSM-V. *American Journal of Psychiatry, 166*, 645–650.

Rhebergen, D., van der Steenstraten, I. M., Sunderland, M., de Graaf, R., Ten Have M., Lamers, F., … Andrews, G. (2014). An examination of generalized anxiety disorder and dysthymic disorder by latent class analysis. *Psychological Medicine, 44*, 1701–1712.

Rimer, J., Dwan, K., Lawlor, D. A., Grieg, C. A., McMurdo, M., Morley, W., & Mead, G. E. (2012). Exercise for depression. *Cohrane Collaboration Library, 7*, CD004366.

Robichaud, M. (2013). Cognitive behaviour therapy targeting intolerance of uncertainty: application to a clinical case of generalized anxiety disorder. *Cognitive and Behavioural Practice, 20*, 251–263.

Robichaud, M. & Dugas, M. J. (2005). Negative problem orientation (part I): psychometric properties of a new measure. *Behaviour Research and Therapy, 43*, 391–401.

Robins, E. & Guze, S. B. (1970). Establishment of diagnostic validity in psychiatric illness: its application to schizophrenia. *Journal of Abnormal Psychology, 110*, 413–422.

Robinson, E., Titov, N., Andrews, G., McIntyre, K., Schwencke, G., & Solley, K. (2010). Internet treatment for generalized anxiety disorder: a randomized controlled trial comparing clinician vs. technician assistance. *PLoS ONE, 5*, e10942.

Roemer, L., Lee, J. K., Salters-Pedneault, K., Erisman, S. M., Orsillo, S. M., & Mennin, D. S. (2009). Mindfulness and emotion regulation difficulties in generalized anxiety disorder: preliminary evidence for independent and overlapping contributions. *Behaviour Therapy, 40*, 142–154.

Roemer, L., Molina, S., & Borkovec, T. D. (1997). An investigation of worry content among generally anxious individuals. *Journal of Nervous Mental Disease, 185*, 314–319.

Roemer, L. & Orsillo, S. M. (2002). Expanding our conceptualization of and treatment for generalized anxiety disorder: integrating mindfulness/acceptance-based approaches with existing cognitive behavioural models. *Clinical Psychology: Science and Practice, 9*, 54–68.

Roemer, L. & Orsillo, S. M. (2007). An open trial of an acceptance-based behaviour therapy for generalized anxiety disorder. *Behaviour Therapy, 38*, 72–85.

Roemer, L., Orsillo, S. M., & Salters-Pedneault, K. (2008). Efficacy of an acceptance-based behaviour therapy for generalized anxiety disorder: evaluation in a randomized controlled trial. *Journal of Consulting and Clinical Psychology, 76*, 1083–1089.

Rosen, N. O. & Knäuper, B. (2009). A little uncertainty goes a long way: state and trait differences in uncertainty interact to increase information seeking but also increase worry. *Health Communication, 24*, 228–238.

Ruscio, A., Borkovec, T. D., & Ruscio, J. (2001). A taxometric investigation of the latent structure of worry. *Journal of Abnormal Psychology, 110*, 413–422.

Ruscio, A., Lane, M., Roy-Byrne, P., Stang, P., Stein, D. J., Wittchen, H. -U., & Kessler, R. C. (2005). Should excessive worry be required for a diagnosis of generalized anxiety disorder? Results from the US National Comorbidity Survey Replication. *Psychological Medicine, 35*, 1761–1772.

Ruscio, A. M. & Borkovec, T. D. (2004). Experience and appraisal of worry among high worriers with and without generalized anxiety disorder. *Behaviour Research and Therapy, 42*, 1469–1482.

Sachdev, P. S., Andrews, G., Hobbs, M. J., Sunderland, M., & Anderson, T. M. (2009). Neurocognitive disorders: cluster 1 of the proposed meta-structure for DSM-V. *Psychological Medicine, 39*, 2001–2012.

Salzer, S., Winkelbach, C., Leweke, F., Leibing, E., & Leichsenring, F. (2011). Long-term effects of short-term psychodynamic psychotherapy and cognitive-behavioural therapy in generalized anxiety disorder: 12-month follow-up. *Canadian Journal of Psychiatry, 56*, 503–508.

Sanderson, W. C. and Barlow, D. H. (1990). A description of patients diagnosed with DSM-III-R generalized anxiety disorder. *Journal of Nervous Mental Disorders, 178*, 588–591.

Shores, M. M., Glubin, T., Cowley, D. S., Dagger, S. R., Roy-Byrne, P., & Dunner, D. L. (1992). The relationship between anxiety and depression: a clinical comparison of generalized anxiety disorder, dysthymic disorder, panic disorder, and major depressive disorder. *Comprehensive Psychiatry, 33*, 237–244.

Siev, J. & Chambless, D. L. (2007). Specificity of treatment effects: cognitive therapy and relaxation for generalized anxiety and panic disorders. *Journal of Consulting and Clinical Psychology, 75*, 513–522.

Slade, T. & Andrews, G. (2001). DSM-IV and ICD-10 generalized anxiety disorder: discrepant diagnoses and associated disability. *Social Psychiatry and Psychiatric Epidemiology, 36*, 45–51.

Slade, T., Johnston, A., Oakley Browne, M. A., Andrews, G., & Whiteford, H. (2009). 2007 National Survey of Mental Health and Wellbeing: methods and key findings. *Australian and New Zealand Journal of Psychiatry, 43*, 594–605.

Slade, T. & Watson, D. (2006). The structure of common DSM-IV and ICD-10 mental disorder in the Australian general population. *Psychological Medicine, 36,* 1593–1600.

Spitzer, R. L., Kroenke, K., Williams, J. B. W., & Löwe, B. (2006). A brief measure for assessing generalized anxiety disorder: the GAD-7. *Archives of Internal Medicine, 166,* 1092–1097.

Stapinski, L. A., Abbott, M. J., & Rapee, R. M. (2010). Evaluating the cognitive avoidance model of generalized anxiety disorder: impact of worry on threat appraisal, perceived control and anxious arousal. *Behaviour Research and Therapy, 48,* 1032–1040.

Starvcevic, V. & Bogojevic, G. . (1999). The concept of generalized anxiety disorder: between the too narrow and the too wide diagnostic criteria. *Psychopathology, 32,* 5–11.

Stöber, J. (1998). Reliability and validity of two widely used worry questionnaires: self-report and self-peer convergence. *Personality and Individual Differences, 24,* 887–890.

Teesson, M., Slade, T., & Mills, K. (2009). Comorbidity in Australia: findings of the 2007 National Survey of Mental Health and Wellbeing. *Australian and New Zealand Journal of Psychiatry, 43,* 606–614.

Thayer, J. F., Friedman, B. H., & Borkovec, T. D. (1996). Autonomic characteristics of generalized anxiety disorder and worry. *Biological Psychiatry, 39,* 255–266.

Titov, N., Andrews, G., Robinson, E., Schwencke, G., Johnston, L., Solley, K., & Choi, I. (2009). Clinician-assisted internet-based treatment is effective for generalized anxiety disorder: a randomized controlled trial. *Australian and New Zealand Journal of Psychiatry, 43,* 905–912.

Titov, N., Dear, B. F., Schwencke, G., Andrews, G., Johnston, L., Craske, M., & McEvoy, P. M. (2011). Transdiagnostic internet treatment for anxiety and depression: a randomized controlled trial. *Behaviour Research and Therapy, 49,* 441–452.

Treanor, M., Erisman, S. M., Salters-Pedneault, K., Roemer, L., & Orsillo, S. M. (2011). Acceptance-based behavioural therapy for GAD: effects on outcomes from three theoretical models. *Depression and Anxiety, 28,* 127–136.

Üstun, T. B. & Sartorius, N. (1995). *Mental illness in general care: an international study.* Chister, NY: Wiley.

van der Heiden, C., Muris, P., & van der Molen, H. T. (2012). Randomized controlled trial on the effectiveness of metacognitive therapy and the intolerance of uncertainty therapy for generalized anxiety disorder. *Behaviour Research and Therapy, 50,* 100–109.

Vollebergh, W. A., Iedema, J., Bijl, R. V., de Graaf, R., Smit, F., & Ormel, J. (2001). The structure and stability of common mental disorders: the NEMESIS study. *Archives of General Psychiatry, 58,* 597–603.

Wang, P. S., Berglund, P., Olfson, M., Pincus, H. A., Wells, K. B., & Kessler, R. C. (2005). Failure and delay in initial treatment contact after first onset of mental disorders in the National Comorbidity Survey Replication. *Archives of General Psychiatry, 62*, 603–613.

Waters, A. M. & Craske, M. G. (2005). Generalized anxiety disorder. In M. M. Anthony, D. R. Ledley, & R. G. Heimberg (Eds.), *Improving outcomes and preventing relapse in cognitive-behavioural therapy*. New York: The Guilford Press.

Watkins, E. R., Moulds, M., & Mackintosh, B. (2005). Comparisons between rumination and worry in a non-clinical population. *Behaviour Research and Therapy, 43*, 1577–1585.

Wells, A. (1995). Meta-cognition and worry: a cognitive model of generalized anxiety disorder. *Behavioural and Cognitive Psychotherapy, 23*(3), 301–320.

Wells, A. (1997). *Cognitive therapy of anxiety disorders: a practice manual and conceptual guide*. Chichester, UK: Wiley.

Wells, A. (1999). A metacognitive model and therapy for generalized anxiety disorder. *Clinical Psychology and Psychotherapy, 6*, 86–95.

Wells, A. (2005a). The metacognitive model of GAD: assessment of meta-worry and relationship with DSM-IV generalized anxiety disorder. *Cognitive Therapy and Research, 29*(1), 107–121.

Wells, A. (2005b). Detached mindfulness in cognitive therapy: a metacognitive analysis and ten techniques. *Journal of Rational Emotive and Cognitive Behaviour Therapy, 23*, 337–355.

Wells, A. & Carter, C. (1999). Preliminary tests of a cognitive model of generalized anxiety disorder. *Behaviour Research and Therapy, 37*, 585–594.

Wells, A. & Carter, K. (2001). Further tests of a cognitive model of generalized anxiety disorder: metacognitions and worry in GAD, panic disorder, social phobia, depression, and non-patients. *Behaviour Therapy, 32*, 85–102.

Wells, A. & Cartwright-Hatton, S. (2004). A short form of the metacognitions questionnaire: properties of the MCQ-30. *Behaviour Research and Therapy, 42*, 385–396.

Wells, A. & Davies, M. (1994). The thought control questionnaire: a measure of individual differences in the control of unwanted thought. *Behaviour Research and Therapy, 32*, 871–878.

Wells, A. & King, P. (2006). Metacognitive therapy for generalized anxiety disorder: an open trial. *Journal of Behaviour Therapy and Experimental Psychiatry, 37*, 206–212.

Wells, A., Welford, M., King, P., Papageorgiou, C., Wisely, J., & Mendel, E. (2010). A pilot randomized trial of metacognitive therapy vs applied relaxation in the treatment of adults with generalized anxiety disorder. *Behaviour Research and Therapy, 48*, 429–434.

Westra, H. A., Arkowitz, H., & Dozois, D. J. (2009). Adding a motivational interviewing pretreatment to cognitive behavioural therapy for generalized anxiety disorder: a preliminary randomized controlled trial. *Journal of Anxiety Disorders*, *23*, 1106–1117.

Wilamowska, Z. A., Thompson-Hollands, J., Fairholme, C. P., Ellard, K. K., Farchione, T. J., & Barlow, D. H. (2010). Conceptual background, development, and preliminary data from the unified protocol for transdiagnostic treatment of emotional disorders. *Depression and Anxiety, 27*, 882–890.

Williams, J. B. W., Gibbon, M., First, M. B., Spitzer, R. L., Davis, M., Borus, J., … Wittchen, H. -U. (1992). The Structured Clinical Interview for DSM-III-R (SCID): II. Multisite test–retest reliability. *Archives of General Psychiatry, 49*, 630–636.

Wittchen, H. -U. (2002). Generalized anxiety disorder: prevalence, burden and cost to society. *Depression and Anxiety, 16*, 162–171.

Wittchen, H.-U., Carter, R. M., Pfister, H., Montgomery, S. A., & Kessler, R. C. (2000). Disabilities and quality of life in pure and comorbid generalized anxiety disorder and major depression in a national survey. *International Clinical Psychopharmacology 15*, 319–328.

Wittchen, H.-U., Lachner, G., Wunderlich, U., & Pfister, H. (1998). Test–retest reliability of the computerised DSM-IV version of the Muchich-Composite International Diagnostic Interview (M-CIDI). *Social Psychiatry and Psychiatric Epidemiology, 33*, 568–578.

Wittchen, H.-U., Nelson, C. B., & Lachner, G. (1998). Prevalence of mental disorders and psychosocial impairments in adolescents and young adults. *Psychological Medicine, 28*, 109–126.

Wittchen, H.-U., Zhao, S., & Kessler, R. C. (1994). DSM-III-R generalized anxiety disorder in the National Comorbidity Survey. *Archives of General Psychiatry, 51*, 335–364.

Wright, A., Krueger, R. F., Hobbs, M. J., Markon, K. E., Eaton, N. R., & Slade, T. (2013). The structure of psychopathology: toward an expanded quantitative empirical model. *Journal of Abnormal Psychology, 122*, 281–294.

Yonkers, K. A., Bruce, S. E., Dyck, I. R., & Keller, M. B. (2003). Chronicity, relapse and illness. Course of panic disorder, social phobia and generalized anxiety disorder: findings in men and women from 8 years of follow-up. *Depression and Anxiety, 17*, 173–179.

Zanarini, M. C., Skodol, A. E., Bender, D., Dolan, R., Sanislow, C., Schaefer, E., … Gunderson, J. G. (2000). The Collaborative Longitudinal Personality Disorders Study: reliability of Axis I and II diagnoses. *Journal of Personality Disorders, 14*, 291–299.

Zbozinek, T. D., Rose, R. D., Wolitzky-Taylor, K. B., Sherbourne, C., Sullivan, G., Stein, M. B., … Craske, M. G. (2012). Diagnostic overlap of generalized anxiety disorder and major depressive disorder in a primary care sample. *Depression and Anxiety, 29*, 1065–1071.

Index